THE Bloodless War OF THE MIND

PART ONE

The product of gene manipulation; *was it a success*?

DR OKWUN OJAH

ISBN: 978-1-922354-61-7 (paperback)

Published in Australia by Dr Okwun Ojah and InHouse Publishing.
www.inhousepublishing.com.au

Printed in Australia by InHouse Print & Design.

INHOUSE PTY LTD PUBLISHING

Acknowledgement

1. Jan Peters "www.absoluteproof.com.au"- Proofreader and Editor.
2. James and Ann Loder of Loder's Computers – Narrabri NSW Australia.
3. Doctors and Nurses of Narrabri District Hospital, Narrabri NSW Australia.

Dedicated to

My wife - Helen, children - Mary-Cynthia, Ral, Colin and Angel,
the Staff Members of my Clinic, especially Jo Parkes –
of Narrabri Medical Centre NSW Australia,
for all their love and support.

Author's Profile

Novelist – Author of the medical thrillers – "It Never Rained; It Poured" published in 2015 and available worldwide. This is my second novel.

Medical Practitioner – Family Physician/GP with interest in Obstetrics.

I have delivered over 3,000 babies in my life as a GP/Obstetrician. Still delivering. Have a peep into my "Babies Wall of Fame" in my Clinic.

Legal Practitioner – Although I hold several degrees (LLB, Grad Dip in Legal Practices, LLM – with Merits) from Australian Universities in Law – , I only attend to medico-legal matters which most often would be writing letters and vetting written letters. I'm extremely busy delivering babies.

Forensic Physician – I hold a diploma in Forensic Medicine from Monash University. I refer to myself as a Forensic Clinician so I attend to "Injuries sustained by life people". I do not enjoy attending to dead bodies.

Bush Doctor – I have successfully ran two Practices in the small town of Narrabri NSW for over 10 years. I am still doing it and still a bush doctor!

I'm a Fellow of:

- Royal Australian College of GP
- Australian College of Rural and Remote Medicine, and
- Australasian College of Legal Medicine.
- I also hold a diploma with Australia Institute of Dermatology.

Philanthropist – I have been extending a helping hand to the rural parts of Eastern Nigerian, Africa where my roots emanate from. See my Charity Website for information on this "Ojah Family Foundation".

Contents

Acknowledgement........................ iii
Dedication.............................. v
Author's Profile vii

Chapter 1 1
Chapter 2 9
Chapter 3 17
Chapter 4 27
Chapter 5 37
Chapter 6 47
Chapter 7 57
Chapter 8 67
Chapter 9 77
Chapter 10..............................87
Chapter 11..............................97
Chapter 12.............................109
Chapter 13.............................119
Epilogue...............................129

Chapter 1

No 30 O'Leary Avenue
Bloemfontein, Orange Free State
South Africa
April 13, 1986, Sunday Morning

Sammy's large body moved restlessly and uncomfortably in his deep sleep and was prevented from falling off their queen-size bed by Abigail. He occupied literally three quarters of the bed leaving the rest for Abigail. Outside their house, the angry storm roared fiercely, and rain pounded on the zinc tin of their roof, as though it intended to create irreparable holes on it. Further away, the thunder grumbled, and the rain dropped in a rhythmic pattern as if heavily armoured soldiers were reporting for duty.

Sammy suddenly woke up, unsure of what woke him, and his eyes darted straight across to the clock that hung opposite their bed. It was 4.00 am. He shook his head. He had barely slept for four hours. His head was pounding, and his eyes were sore. He felt as though he had not slept at all. His eyes were closed but his mind was wide awake. He knew he would not be able to sleep well anymore, not now, and not in the near future. His mind was full of weird thoughts; some were enough to cause children to have nightmares, and his eyes were heavy and achy with insomnia. He had not slept well for the past three days since Manly passed away.

With the back of his hand, he wiped away the tears that were rolling down his cheeks and obliterating his vision. As he did that, his eyes strayed to the far end of the room where a structure caught his attention.

Through his foggy sight, all he could see were the withering and wilting plants, but he quickly scanned beyond the pots on the floor and up the wall where the picture hung. He quietly extricated himself from the bed so as not to disturb Abigail and made his way across to the picture.

And he stared at it, 'Father, why did you have to go so soon? What will I do now without you? Who will I look up to? Who will advise me?' He sobbed and asked the same questions over and over again, and could not take his eyes away from his late father's photo in its ornate frame. He gazed intensely at it till he could see no more.

"Only the Divine Creator could answer all your questions, darling." Abigail responded from behind him, with tears flowing from her own eyes.

Sammy turned and looked at her. She was staring at the opposite wall. Her eyes welled up with such a sadness engulfing her pretty face and making her appear ten times older than her natural age. They seemed to show the ache that was nibbling away at her soul. But wasn't it she who declared to him, "I'll be strong for you," many times since the death of his father?

Peering through his tear-filled eyes, "You're crying too," he uttered and shook his head.

"Hmmm…" was her response. She grabbed her handkerchief, began to dab her face and with heavy feet she sluggishly drifted towards their sofa and sank into it lethargically.

The thought of life without Mighty M, as Manly was fondly known, made Sammy's heart to ache and his body to shake convulsively. Manly was more than a father. He was his role model. The relationship he had with him transcended that of father and son. His father would crack jokes with him as if they were age mates. He taught him all he knew today. He encouraged him to marry Abigail when

Sammy wasn't sure of what he wanted and even lent him money for their wedding. He also raised the deposit for their first home. Sammy could not stop longing for him. Mighty M was a good man who did not deserve death, not the way it happened. He was six-foot-tall and was referred to as a 'gentle giant.' He had a gentle spirit, and he was generous too.

Sammy was still in denial that Mighty M was gone forever.

Neither Sammy, nor Abigail spoke again. Silence crept into their room and engulfed it like a ghost. Sammy sank into the sofa and pulled Abigail towards him. It was six in the morning and eerily quiet except for the pitter patter of the rain. Birds would usually be singing by this time, but not today. It seemed that they were too cold to sing. His neighbours all seemed to have taken sleeping pills, there was no sign of life outside. Nobody was preparing for church. There wasn't even a hoot or screech of a car in the street.

With the handkerchief on her face, "So when will he ... ?" Abigail muttered but couldn't complete the sentence.

"Do you mean when will he be buried?" Sammy completed the question for her.

"Yeah," she continued to sob.

"We'll see Uncle Goddy tomorrow, to find out if the elders have met and discussed his burial."

"How long can he be left in the morgue?"

"It depends on what the elders have decided," he responded in a melancholic voice.

"Is your mum still in their house?"

He stole a glance at her, "Are you asking if they've taken her away?"

"I would've thought so given that your father died in that house." She frowned. "Our culture requires widows to leave the house immediately after their husband is pronounced dead. The exit time is quicker if the death happened at home." She paused. "When my uncle died, my auntie was whisked away in less than 30 minutes after his death."

"My mum is with Uncle Goddy now." Sammy slowly looked up and down at the ceiling with baggy eyes.

Abigail leaned on to Sammy's shoulder, "Can I make you a cup of coffee?"

"I wouldn't mind," he responded with his face cupped in his hands and in tears.

As Abigail stood and began to walk to the kitchen, the phone rang.

"Please can you grab it," Sammy asked? "Put it on speaker."

As it was barely 7.00 am; Abigail wondered who would be ringing them so early in the morning.

"Hello, Abigail Petters speaking."

"Hello Abbie, it's me – Michael Petters, your brother-in-law in Australia."

"Hello, Mikky. How's Sydney?" Abigail replied and beckoned Sammy to come on over.

"It's still cold here."

"I'll get your brother to talk to you as I'm heading to the kitchen to do something," she told him and continued on her way.

Sammy stood up immediately and walked over to the phone, "Is that you Mikky, my brother?"

"Yeah, it's me..."

"How's Agnes, your wife?"

"She's okay," he responded in a very subdued tone.

Michael then began to cry loudly, making convulsive gasps. Sammy began also. They both continued wailing till they had no strength left in them.

Abigail heard what was going on and walked back with two cups of coffee in her hands, "Mikky and Sammy, we all have to start holding ourselves together."

Shortly after saying that, she began to bawl also.

Sammy turned around and noticed that his wife is crying. He stopped and wiped tears away from her face, and then dried his own. "Is Agnes there with you now?"

"Yeah, I am," Agnes responded. "How's my sister-in-law Abbie?"

Abigail took over from her husband who was yet to regain his composure. "I could have said I'm great, but the death of Mighty M has left me devastated and very sad."

"It's done the same to us over here," Agnes chipped in. "Mikky and I have not slept since we got the news yesterday."

"What time is it now, in Australia?"

"6.00 pm," Agnes replied soberly.

Michael came back online, "Sammy, how did it happen?"

"Do you mean how did dad die?" Sammy quizzed him.

"Yeah, the phone was not clear when Uncle Goddy rang to inform us of his death."

Sammy took a deep breath, and shifted a few times on his chair before beginning to explain.

"He died in the bathtub, while taking his bath," he sighed.

"Do you mean he had a fit while in the bathtub?" Michael asked?

"Pretty much, yeah," his brother replied.

Sammy went on to narrate, "Each epileptic attack he had, ended up being prolonged and the doctors called it status epilepticus. In the last few months of his life he was having seizures three times every week. It became difficult for him to lead a meaningful life."

Michael interjected, "So he even resigned from the Mines and stopped going to his farm?"

"Despite how much he loved his work and the farm, he had to give them both up and mum had to tend to everything from then," Sammy stated. "Indeed, he lost his will to live. He literally stopped existing."

Apologetic for interrupting Abigail stated, "I sensed it was a huge problem when he also had to give up his licence and stop driving."

"So who drove him around?" Agnes inquired.

"My mother-in-law," Abigail responded. "As you know, she is not confident with driving and hates doing it at the best of times, but she was compelled to do so."

"From the look of things, he should've been monitored during all activities, especially when he took his bath, am I right?" Michael asked.

"Yeah, you are," Sammy agreed, and went on to offer further explanation. "It seems that mum went out to buy some groceries on that day and it appears that dad then decided to hop into the bathtub, as it was pretty hot. The result was that he had a seizure that claimed his life while in the bathtub."

"It's a sad event," Michael ejaculated. Agnes made a similar sound to register her acquiescence without uttering any audible word.

"You're absolutely correct," Sammy responded.

Abigail shook her head in sadness, "That's where the problem lay; it was difficult to provide Mighty M with 24-hour round the clock care. It only took a fraction of a second for the disaster to strike. Who would've imagined that he would've drowned in his own bathtub?"

"So, who found him?" Agnes queried.

"It was mum," Sammy said. "When she came back that afternoon from the shops she found him face down in the bathtub. His towel and undies were lying on the bathroom floor. According to mum she knew immediately that dad had suffered another status epilepticus." He paused and took a breath.

Michael and his wife were keen to hear more of the story.

Abigail then took over the story telling, "His fits according to your mum had become very frequent, and it seemed they were becoming drug resistant and more prolonged. From what your mother told us, he had stopped attending his doctors' appointments because in his language, the doctors' treatment had failed him."

"What a life!" Sammy sounded exasperated. "The doctors guessed that his epilepsy was in his genes, but they were neither able to find out what actually caused it, nor were they able to cure him, and that made him despair."

"So he gave up?" Michael suggested.

"It appears so," Sammy affirmed. "To make matters worse all the drugs that they prescribed for him gave him significant side effects and that prompted him to become non-compliant."

"It would've been a dreadful sight for your mother to see, him lying face down in the bathtub," Agnes opined.

Abigail agreed, "It's awful. She told me that she screamed at the top of her lungs when she saw him. Luckily she'd come back home with her friend – Lucy Jackman. It was Lucy who called the ambulance and informed Sammy."

It seemed Sammy had recovered a bit, so he could continue narrating the events. "Immediately dad stopped taking his medications mother feared that she would lose him to epilepsy and her fears became real on that fateful day."

Michael heaved and sighed. "We'll be booking our flight later today and we'll put in for probably two to three months leave." He paused.

"Yeah we'll do that," Agnes confirmed.

"When do you think that you will arrive home?" Sammy questioned.

"We'll fly in tomorrow. And we'll all meet at Uncle Goddy's house."

"See you guys tomorrow," Sammy and Abigail wished Michael and Agnes a safe flight.

Sammy knows that his younger brother is very reliable. Although he's two years his junior, Michael is physically stronger than him and handles stress a lot better. They love each other and have an intimate relationship. He can't wait to see him. He usually leans on Michael's shoulder when he's in need and he certainly needs him now more than ever before.

Shortly after Michael and Agnes hung up, the phone rang again.

Sammy beckoned his wife, "Darling, please answer the phone and put it on speaker so that we can both join in the conversation."

Abigail grabbed the phone, "Hello, who's on the line?"

"It's me Nancy, is that you Abbie?"

"Yeah, how are you? Your brother's here."

"How're you Nancy?" Sammy joined in.

"I'm okay although very sad."

"Where are you now?" Sammy asked.

"I'm driving to Pretoria to see Uncle Goddy and I understand that mama is with him. Am I right?"

"Yeah that's the information that we've got too," Sammy replied.

"What's your plan?" asked Nancy.

"Abigail and I will be heading that way tomorrow."

"So, I'll see you guys there," Nancy said.

"Sure, see you there too," Sammy enjoined.

He has never had a cosy relationship with his elder sister. Although she is only two years his senior, they never really had any attachment, call it bond, between them since they were little. To make matters worse she decided to go into modelling rather than to settle down like other young ladies of her age. She was also a drop-out from high school. It seems like she doesn't enjoy having any lengthy discussions with Sammy, and vice-versa. They usually speak in monosyllables. However, they never actually engaged each other in any physical fight. They'll complete their discussion in Pretoria.

Chapter 2

Sammy's Cadillac Model 30
Orange Free State Highway
South Africa
April 14, 1986, Monday Morning

When Sammy and Abigail stepped out of their house, sunlight had filled the sky. The clouds had become beautified with a spectrum of colours and blue tinges which ambitiously illuminated every crevice of the land. Birds were singing an explicit background melody and the trees were dancing under the chilly autumn wind. The breeze was soothing and calming but not enough as to quell the anguish that tormented Sammy and his wife. Gazing upwards to the illuminated sky and clouds, Abigail felt at home in a way she never had before, but Sammy didn't.

"Shall we make a start? We've got to be in Pretoria by 4.00 pm today," Sammy urged his wife who had rushed back into the house to pick up her purse and other personal effects.

"I'll be out soon. I've found it," Abigail sang out from inside.

Some minutes later, Abigail came out and they got in their car and drove off.

As Sammy revved his favourite Cadillac, a Model 30, along the N1 highway, the noise from it was deafening. The car's exhaust pipe chucked out brownish thick toxic fumes that recoiled through the open roof and back into the car. Abigail had to cover her nostrils with her handkerchief so as not to inhale the carbon monoxide fumes. Sammy was speeding and he seemed to be enjoying it. Abigail knows he loves to speed. He sped to bury his sorrows. He also had the music of Yvonne Chaka Chaka on. He loved the musician as much as he loved his 1975 Cadillac. Abigail thinks that the music tends to send him into a speeding frenzy. His speeding habit has recently earned him the name of "a speed demon" amongst his friends.

Abigail pointed to the dashboard, "Darling, you're doing 140km/hr in a zone of 120."

Sammy immediately glanced at his speedometer. "I'm sorry." He applied the brake briefly only to accelerate a short while later.

Each time he pressed the accelerator, the car flapped and squealed from underneath, and Abigail cringed. The noise and vibrations continued and reached a zenith that Abigail couldn't tolerate any longer.

"Do you mind slowing down a bit?" Abigail pleaded nervously.

"Why?"

"Because, you are now doing 160km/hr."

Sammy pursed his lips and was slow in responding.

"Do you actually want us to reach Uncle Goddy's place in one piece?" Abigail asked.

"I'm really, really sorry." Sammy was repentant.

Abigail knows he hasn't been himself since his father passed away. She is worried that they might crash and not make it to Pretoria.

"You know my state of mind right now," Sammy murmured. He then reduced the speed again.

"I know exactly how you're feeling." Turning to cast a loving glance at him, Abigail stated emphatically, "I'd hate to have one of us die on this road without making it to Uncle Goddy's house."

"I'll set the cruise control at 120 from now."

Abigail leaned forward and planted a kiss on his cheek. "I love you." As she looked out of the window and observed the brown grasses that appeared to be begging for some moisture and water as well as some sunflowers that nodded in the wind as their speedy car drove past, she lapsed into memory lane...

∞ ∞

Around 10.00 am on July 30, 1985, a day after their wedding, Sammy rang her ...

"I've got something exciting to show you," he blurted out.

"Are you coming home?"

"Yes, right now," he replied.

"Is it another herbal cure from those native doctors?" she queried.

"Calm down, Darl. It's something better than that," he said reassuringly.

She still didn't believe him and wondered what it could be. 'It must certainly have something to do with the cure for his father's status epilepticus attacks?' she convinced herself.

Lately, they have been extremely petrified that Mighty M's epilepsy might be passed on to their unborn children, so she and Sammy have been scavenging for a cure. Sammy practically had been visiting all native herbalists seeking a solution.

On second thought, she picked up her mobile phone and dialled him, "Have you been offered a new job?"

"I'm few minutes away from home. You'll see it when I zoom in," he said with a laugh.

She thought that it could be that he had been offered a new job. He had been out of a job for more than six months. Earlier that year, his new boss fired him. His boss observed that he was unable to bend and kneel for more than 20 minutes while at work and being a mechanic that was very necessary. He was also compelled to take a break every so often to straighten his legs. He, however, hadn't obtained permission to do so from the Management. The new boss wasn't happy with him and sent him a query. Sammy responded to the query and tried to explain to him that he has had a weak right leg and painful hip from childhood. He doesn't know why he has the condition, especially with regard to his hip. Neither the doctors he had visited, nor his parents had been able to explain the cause of the hip pain to him. He took the break in order to contain the pain. His boss wouldn't accept that and fired him. Sammy was so distressed and felt completely helpless until his younger brother stepped in and got a lawyer who took on the case. The lawyer took the case to the Industrial Tribunal and they were still waiting for the outcome.

"So what's the exciting news?" she asked.

"Wait till I get home," was his reply.

It wasn't long before Sammy got home. Upon arriving home he reached for the door knob, twisted and pushed it in quick succession. The door slammed on Abigail's face as she was rushing from inside to open the door to hear the exciting news from her husband.

"Oh, sorry for slamming the door on your face," he apologised.

"I'm not terribly hurt." She smiled at him. "I was coming to meet you and see what the good news is."

He thrust a cheque of R50,000 at her as well as a confirmation letter stating it was a payout for wrongful dismissal. "You see what I meant when I told you, it's exciting news."

Abigail was ecstatic, "You're absolutely correct my darling" and leapt into Sammy's open arms. They had never had such money in their lives.

After the payout they began to discuss how to invest the money. She wanted the money to be put into a fixed deposit and for them to use the accruing interest to buy a house and to open a savings account for their children.

Sammy however had different ideas; he wanted to buy a car he could drive. He had been unable to drive any manual car because of his weak leg and she had been the family chauffeur.

A week later, Sammy came back from the Club on a sunny afternoon clutching a newspaper in his right hand and immediately dropped it on the table in front of Abigail.

"Look at page 20," he said, and pointed at the car advertisement. It read: "A used 1975 model Cadillac, single owner, priced reasonably well, with hand control equipment and devices for people who have limited use of their legs." He paused and looked up at Abigail. "This is for me," he exclaimed ecstatically. He was obviously beside himself with joy.

Abigail hesitated. She slowly walked away from him towards the bedroom.

He tiptoed after her. "Aren't you happy that I've found a car that will suit me?"

"I'm happy for you and probably for us. The devil is in the detail. What is this car going to cost us?"

"The advert states – price negotiable," Sammy advised.

"Remember, I'll want us to start saving for our own home as well as for our kids' schooling."

She reluctantly shared in her husband's joy; her fear being that she did not want them spending the whole payout money on the car.

Sammy scratched his goatee beard. "Let's sit down and discuss this thoroughly."

Immediately she sat down, and he sat beside her. "You're correct; we need a house and savings for our unborn children." He paused.

Abigail had frown lines on her face. "So, how're we going to achieve our aim if you're to plough all the money into this car?"

"Let's say we aim to spend a maximum of R30,000 on the car and then you can take the rest to start up a business from which we can start saving for our home. We'll aim to save for kids later, probably, when they're born. How does that sound?"

Since her attempt at dissuading him has failed she really has to accept the deal he has proposed. "Okay, let's go for the car."

Sammy hugged and kissed her.

The next day, they attended Monsumi's Exotic Car Dealers on the East Rand where the Cadillac car was housed. A fast-talking car dealer by the name Abraham attended to them that day.

Focusing on her, Abraham said, "You see, your husband limps slightly on his right leg, so he can't drive a manual or automatic car that has foot pedals. He needs a special car fitted with hand-controlled levers. He needs this Cadillac. It is the ultimate driving machine. It has class. You will never regret it once you have driven in it. Besides the devices are installed in such a way that both of you can drive it."

"How will we achieve that?" she remembered asking him.

"The pedals are located both on the floor and on the steering wheel. A device is installed on the steering wheel and operated using a small lever with the thumb."

"Will there be a button that can be added for cruise control?" she remembered asking.

"Yes," he replied and added, "On the alternative the accelerator rings could be attached either over the top of, or behind the existing steering wheel, and for the car to accelerate these need to be pushed or pulled against the steering wheel. Sammy could choose any device that appealed to him the most.

He looked at them and concluded, "The floor pedals will be for you Madam and the steering for your husband." He flashed his well cleaned whitish set of dentures.

At that point, Sammy whispered into her ear, "Let's go for the car, I'm in love with it."

They asked for the car registration papers which they inspected, and Sammy signed, transferring ownership to them.

Abraham then led them into the workshop to see the modification specialist.

Both the cost of the car and the equipment installation totalled R 29,500. ..

∞ ∞

A loud noise on the windscreen jarred Abigail back to reality. "Was that a bird that just flew into our windscreen?" she asked her husband.

"Yes, it was. And the poor bird died instantly," he stated satirically.

"A bird hitting your car windscreen really is an omen of death," Abigail commented.

"It's a fluke. I don't believe in that," Sammy responded. "Even if it's real, we already have a death in the family, which it could have symbolised."

Abigail is getting concerned that Sammy is pressing down on the accelerator very hard and very fast. They have had this discussion that he should reduce his speed a lot lately.

With a twisted face, Abigail hinted, "You're doing more than 120km/hr again."

"Is that so," Sammy asked almost absentmindedly. "I didn't know."

"Why would you know when you are so engrossed with Yvonne Chaka Chaka's music?"

"It isn't the music, rather the location of the accelerator on my hands that makes it easy for the car to speed up. What's more her music helps to calm me down."

"Oh, does it?" Abigail asked ironically.

Sammy turned and looked at his lovely wife and chuckled. "You're jealous, ain't you?"

"You're practising love through telepathy, ain't you?" Abigail replied.

They both shrugged it off.

Abigail dislikes Yvonne and her music because Sammy likes both the lady and her music immensely. He attends all her concerts and performances. He once confessed while attending Yvonne's concert with Abigail, that he had a huge crush on Yvonne and would do anything to reach her if given a chance. Abigail felt unappreciated and disappointed. That was when the seed of hatred was sewn in her mind. She took solace in the fact that Sammy was so faithful that he would never actually do anything to hurt her. However, given that she felt hurt, she brought up the topic with Sammy the next day.

When confronted Sammy denied making such a comment. However, he owned up when Amanda, a friend who also attended the concert with them, confirmed it. He apologised to Abigail and blamed the alcohol as the reason for the comment. He then declared his unfaltering love for Abigail and bought her presents. He did not promise not to attend future Yvonne Chaka Chaka's shows and for her part, Abigail was not entirely convinced that he was not infatuated with the musician. She decided not to pursue the matter any further. However, it rips her heart apart whenever she sees him watching and dancing to Yvonne Chaka Chaka's musics.

"We're at Kempton Park." Sammy slowed down and brought the car to a stop at the traffic lights. "We've got less than an hour to reach Hills Street."

"Can we stop at the next fuel station so that I can ease myself?" Abigail suggested.

"I'll need to refill the car and ease myself too," Sammy indicated as he slowed and steered into the FlyBuy Petrol station.

Abigail had obvious admiration for the scenery of Kempton Park. Although her parents were from Botswana, they once lived in Kempton Park and she was born there. She attended the primary school at Shangari-La Academy before relocating to Pretoria where she attended high school and completed her university degree. Her parents and her sister, Bianca still live in Sandton city which is the next suburb to Kempton Park.

As they were walking back to their car, Abigail tapped Sammy on the arm, "Darling we forgot to buy some wine."

Sammy threw his arm around her. "That's not a problem; probably we'll have to drive to Greenstone Shopping Mall in Jo'burg." He glanced at her. "Does that suit you?"

"That's great." She smiled. "I'll grab some cloths for Tiny while we're there."

Chapter 3

Sammy's Cadillac Model 30
Kempton Park roads and Johannesburg Highway
South Africa
April 14, 1986, Monday Evening

With her legs crossed and her knees resting on the car's dashboard, Abigail watched Sammy stoop low, slide into the driver's seat and starting the engine with the push of a button. As she watched him, she had the desire to touch him and run her fingers through his beard and caress him. She resisted the urge because they were in the car and had an urgent mission to accomplish. She quickly withdrew her hands and rather, began rubbing them together.

Observing Abigail's movements, Sammy read her mind, and decided to stop briefly before driving into the main street from the Fuel Station. He then bent sideways to plant his lips on hers. Before their faces could come together, they heard a loud bump from their rear and their car lunged forward.

Sammy had an angry frown on his face, and looked back, "They've run into us," he stated furiously.

As he began to release his seat belt, Abigail grabbed his hand. "Don't get out," she commanded.

Sammy looked at her and she returned his glance. He reapplied his seat belt very fast immediately and started the engine.

As he was waiting for the main street to be car free so as to drive off, he cast a glance at his rear vision mirror and observed the driver of the car waving at him.

"Is he saying that he's sorry?" Abigail asked.

"It seems so."

"Do you believe him?" she asked.

"No." Sammy turned and looked at Abigail. "Where's your mobile phone?"

"In my handbag."

"Grab it and ring the police."

As Abigail bent down to grab her phone, Sammy gave further orders, "Don't elevate it to the level that the guys in that car will see it."

Abigail took her phone and keeping it on top of her handbag, pressed the speaker knob and then dialled the police number.

"Hello, this is Constable Kagiso from Johannesburg Central Police Station."

"Hello Constable, I'm Abigail Petters. I'm in the car with my husband – Sammy. We suspect that we've got car snatchers tail-gating us as I speak."

"Where are you people now?"

"Just driving off from Flybuy Petrol Station in Kempton Park and heading to Jo'burg."

"Tell me a bit more," Constable Kagiso requested.

"They bumped into our car just as we were about to drive onto the street from the petrol station." She paused then continued. "They intended for us to jump out of our car to see if there's any damage then they would pounce and hijacked our car."

"Okay," Constable replied. "Please, describe the car."

"It's a black Toyota Corolla Quest car, and it looks like it's a 1980 model."

"Can you make out its plate number and its occupants?"

Sammy joined in the phone discussion immediately. "The plate number is covered. There are three of them, two in the front and one in the back seat."

“I’m on my way with my team to you right now,” Constable Kagiso advised. “Where are you now?”

“We’ve driven through Kelvin Street and CR Swart Drive, just about to enter Pretoria Road from there we aim to go onto the R102 Highway.” Abigail added.

“Are they still following you?”

“They were initially two cars behind us while we were at Kelvin Street and CR Swart Drive. They’re now a car behind us.” Sammy heaved a big sigh.

“We’ll likely meet you people at the R102 Highway. Be careful on that highway as it is thehotspot for car snatchers.

“Is that so?” Abigail enquired.

“Yes,” the Constable replied. “Keep your phone on and give me a running commentary of their moves.”

“We’ll do so,” Sammy responded.

“Be careful, do not allow them to overtake you at any time or they may shoot you,” the Constable advised them.

“How soon will you meet us?” Abigail asked with a quivering voice.

“Where’re you people now?” Constable asked.

“We are just entering the R102 Highway now,” Sammy responded.

“Are they still following you?”

With tears in her eyes, Abigail replied, “Yes, and they’re trying to overtake us.”

“Sammy, be brave, don’t let them overtake you,” the Constable encouraged him. “My team and I’ve entered the North end of the R102 Highway.”

“Thanks, I’m okay,” Sammy replied with a brave face.

Fright and terror pierced through Sammy’s soul, but none made it to his face. His hand remained steady on the steering as if he was relaxing with a novel. His fear was only displayed on the speed range he was making.

According to Constable Kagiso, it seems that the rule of engagement for hijackers is to shoot after they've overtaken the victim and more so if the person refuses to surrender. Sammy's target will be not to allow them to overtake him. So far, so good, he's ahead of them. But whenever they draw closer, his heart skips a beat and his breathe becomes shallower. Whatever is the case, the present task is to remain composed. He has to meet this fear with the same resistance a rock shows to wind. Having resolved to win he has to let his fear blow around him.

On the other hand, Abigail is wet with sweat. Her clothes are soaked from her underwear to the skirt and blouse on the outside. Her eyes are hot and throbbing as she is glued to the mirrors and the dashboard. She is literarily gauging the speed of the assailants and encouraging Sammy to go faster. They are racing for their lives. Her heart is thumping heavily against her chest. Her fingers are curled into a fist, and her nails are digging deep into her palms.

Abigail glances at the side mirror then at the dashboard, "Darling, increase your speed, they are drawing closer."

Sammy responded appropriately by accelerating to 160km per hour and overtaking a small 304 Peugeot car, his car skidded a bit as he overtakes the car.

Abigail lets out a deep breath, as a sigh of relief, "That's good they are now two cars behind us again."

Each time Sammy accelerates, the car skids a bit because the road is wet and as slippery as an eel. It had rained a day ago. When the car skids, his hands shake and the steering wobbles. He knows that he has to keep his hands and the steering steady and straight if he is to arrive alive. By law his car must be driven within the white lines. He's determined to do so except if he has to obstruct them from overtaking him, and that's when he will skid over the yellow line.

The roads were built in the days of apartheid when there was significant wealth and grandeur. They are duel carriage and wide enough for several cars on each lane. They were flat, smooth and glossy black when they were built with neat lines of white and yellow. These days they've turned grey, cracked, and pot-holed. These days white paint is still clear and visible whereas the yellow has faded in some areas.

Abigail reluctantly glanced at the side mirror and ejaculated, "They are flashing their headlights."

Sammy briefly scanned the rear mirror and noted that she was correct. "It seems that's another of their tricks to get us to slow down."

"The two cars behind us have slowed down for them and they're overtaking them." Abigail observes.

"These hijackers are employing subtle and murderous tactics to reach us," Sammy responded.

Looking at the mirror again, Abigail sees that the hijackers are fast catching up with them. "Increase your speed and overtake the Mercedes."

Sammy accelerates and overtakes the Mercedes and the hijackers recede to a car behind them again.

The sun has begun to set, and Sammy's visibility had become impaired. He switched on the headlights but it was reflecting on the pools of water on the road and making it more difficult for him to see very much ahead.

Suddenly Abigail screamed, "That's a dead body lying on the road," and pointed some metres ahead of them.

Sammy applied the brakes and swerved so they were able to avoid running over the dead body.

Immediately Sammy slowed down, the hijackers overtook the Mercedes car and caught up with them.

Both Sammy's and the hijackers' cars were now driving neck-and-neck. Sammy wasn't going to let them beat him, he wasn't stopping for anything and he sure as hell wasn't taking his hands off the accelerator.

Abigail glanced at the hijackers but couldn't see any of them clearly. Their windows were heavily tinted. Her eyes were glued to their window. The more she looked the less she saw. Her sight had become blurry. She was, however, happy that they hadn't been shot so far.

She held onto the dashboard squeezing it very hard with clenched fists. Her heart was racing at a speed faster than their car was doing. She could hear her own rapid breathing but couldn't feel oxygen going in and out of her lungs. Her stomach was churning with tense cramps. She closed her eyes tightly hoping that it would end up as a dream. She suddenly felt the hijackers overtaking them and jerked up.

"Don't let them, please," she screamed at Sammy.

Sammy accelerated but wasn't seeing clearly and he knew they would crash if he didn't slow down and at that point knew he had to give up.

Suddenly, one of the hijacker's car window started rolling down, and a hooded male with a gun pointing at them commanded, "Stop or we will blow ya head off."

As Sammy pretended to be stopping, he sped off again. The hijackers began to chase them and at that point fired at them. The bullet hit the back of their car and that caused Sammy's car to swerve and roll, down the side of the highway and landing on its roof inside the bush nearby.

"Are you there?" Sammy cried out to Abigail.

"I think I'm fine," Abigail replied.

Being too scared to crawl out, Abigail curled into Sammy's hand and they both stayed in the car, waiting for what fate had in store for them.

Suddenly they heard the sound of sirens, and when Abigail looked out—the car had blue flickers. It came charging at the hijackers from an adjoining road.

Next thing she heard, "Bang, Bang, Bang," several times. Then she heard the sound of a helicopter landing nearby, and more sounds of sirens.

As the gun shots slowly died down, they heard people discussing their whereabouts. Within a short time they heard footsteps approaching them.

A lady in police uniform eventually got to where Sammy and Abigail were trapped in their car. "Mr and Mrs Petters, are you all right?" the lady asked.

"Yeah, we're alive," replied Sammy.

"Ok, I'll call some of the ambulance men to come and help bring you people out," she advised.

"Thanks for that," Abigail responded.

She then walked back to where the others were and in a short while came back followed by a policeman, and four men who wore ambulance uniform.

The ambulance men and police officers worked arduously and eventually overturned Sammy's car and then proceeded to pull Sammy and Abigail out of it.

Immediately they got out, the helpers began to introduce themselves.

"I'm Sergeant Bet," the lady stated.

"Hello Sergeant Bet," Sammy responded.

Meanwhile it became clear that Abigail was wobbly and unsteady on her feet.

"Bring the ambulance here," Sergeant Bet commanded.

The ambulance vehicle was driven to where they were. A man and a lady climbed out of the vehicle. The man spoke, "I'm Joseph and my colleague is Annitey."

They then encouraged Abigail to climb onto the stretcher and then loaded her into the ambulance where they began to administer first aid treatment to her.

Sammy was however still looking okay and conversing very well.

Sergeant Bet continued with her introduction, "This is Constable Kagiso, my colleague who you spoke to earlier."

Sammy stretched out his hand to Constable Kagiso, "Thanks for all your help."

"You're welcome," he replied.

"Five of us attended this rescue mission. One of us is in the vehicle," Sergeant Bet advised and pointed to the location of their van. "The other two are with the Forensic Team doctors in the secured area."

"How many ambulance people and forensic doctors are here?" Sammy asked.

"I think, there are five forensic doctors, six ambulance men and two plain clothed detectives," Sergeant Bet advised him.

"Thanks to all of you for coming to save us," Sammy replied.

"That's our job, more so you gave us enough information which helped us to come to your aid."

"What happened to them," Sammy asked.

Constable Kagiso took over the discussion, "Two engaged us in a gun battle and they were killed but the driver had no gun and surrendered."

"So, you've got him now?" Sammy inquired.

"Yes, we do. He's in the van and will soon be taken to the Station for interrogation. The dead and their car are in the secured area."

As they were conversing, Abigail walked back to them. "I'm fine. I really don't need to go to the hospital and don't need to be in an ambulance," she commented.

"Are you sure?" Constable Kagiso asked her.

"Yeah, I'm perfectly all right now. I think I had a panic attack."

They all turned to inspect Sammy's car. They noticed a greenish liquid on the ground around the car and inside it. "It seems that the bullet ripped off the fuel tank," Constable Kagiso observed.

"We were lucky that you people came on time. We would've been ablaze with the fuel. They were so angry because we gave them a hard time—they would have ignited the car and burnt us alive," Sammy stated.

"They were very vicious. They could've done anything," Sergeant Bet responded and Constable Kagiso confirmed it. "They had .22 and .38 pistols on them."

Sergeant Bet started retreating, "May I beg to leave now? I'll take you home when you're ready," she announced.

"Sure," Sammy responded.

"Constable Kagiso, did you people retrieve the dead body that was lying on the road?" Abigail asked with interest.

Constable Kagiso was amused, "It wasn't a real person. We inspected it. It appeared to be a dead person but it was in fact, some clothing and bags rolled up to look like a real person. This was another of the tactics that they use to trick people to stop in order to render help to a victim on the road. When someone stops they'll pounce on the person and hijack his car."

At that point Sergeant Bet and some other ambulance men come back.

"We're ready to go," Sergeant Bet announced.

Constable Kagiso approached Sergeant Bet and they had a brief discussion.

"I'll take Mr and Mrs Petters home to Montana Park, Pretoria," she announced. "And Constable Kagiso will tow their car to a repair garage."

Sammy and Abigail shook hands with Constable Kagiso, "Thanks once more for helping us."

"Bye for now. See you guys later," he announced.

Sammy and Abigail marched to the police vehicle and were driven away.

Chapter 4

Prince's Pavilion
7004 Hill Street
Montana Park, Pretoria
South Africa
April 14, 1986, Monday Evening - Night

It was 10.00 pm by the time Sammy and Abigail eventually entered Montana Park from where they headed to Hill Street.

The street was deserted, long, wet and winding. It lay under a blanket of silence with a starry rainbow sky hovering overhead like a multi-coloured sheet over a bed. Apart from the pit-pattering sounds of the rain and the tumbling noise of the water in the gutters on its banks, it was like a ghost town; thanks to the ever-increasing spats of stealing and armed robbery in the area. Birds were singing lullabies that were enough to sedate some of the occupants of the street who were calm enough to doze off. There were short green trees on the sides of the street swaying and dancing as the strong breeze blew around them.

On each side, were houses that were separated by huge and high fences that were fortified with electric wires. They appeared to be competing among themselves for height.

At the entrance of the street was a faded zebra crossing and an unattended traffic light which frantically changed colours like a disco light, and at the west end towards Uncle Goddy's pavilion were a few gates with tents for their watchmen.

As the Police vehicle which was transporting Sammy and Abigail drove past, they observed a watchman in one of the tents whose neck was tilted to the side. He was so deep in slumber and snored so loudly and was quite oblivious to the passing car.

In the 70s, it was a plush neighbourhood in which most of the buildings on this street used to boast more sports cars than would be available in Holly-wood, but not anymore. They now boasted of more high-rising fences than the Maximum Prison of South Africa. House burglary had compelled house owners to replace sports cars with push bikes. The few who could still afford them certainly had money to procure security guards to patrol 24 hours of the day.

As Sammy and Abigail drove through Hill Street, all they could hear was "woof, woof".

"These dogs are really growling angrily at us," Sergeant Bet observed.

"They are howling aggressively so as to scare us away," Sammy commented.

"If anyone dares step closer to these dogs, they will maul the person to shreds," Abigail chipped in.

"You've got to be a criminal to step closer to these vicious animals," Sergeant Bet commented. "Where will I drop you people?"

Sammy scanned around and urged her to continue ahead, "At the end of the street."

Sergeant Bet accelerated slowly and glanced at Sammy for instructions of when to pull over.

Immediately they reached a white mansion, Sammy requested, "Please drop us here."

"Who lives here?" Sergeant Bet asked.

"Uncle Goddy, my dad's older brother," Sammy replied.

"Ok," Constable Bet replied and brought the vehicle to a standstill.

Sammy and Abigail collected the few pieces of luggage they had and hopped out of the vehicle. "Thanks for your help tonight," they said. "We're grateful."

"You're welcome." She informed them with sympathy. "Please take care of yourselves. Try and rest very well tonight."

"We'll do just that," they echoed.

Sergeant Bet handed her business card to Sammy, "We'll expect you at the Station tomorrow for us to obtain full statements." She took a breath and paused briefly, "We may also release your vehicle to you so that you can proceed to the garage for repairs."

Sammy looked at her fixedly as if expecting further clarification.

"I mean as long as our Forensic department have finished with it then we will release it to you," she further advised.

"Fine, we'll be there tomorrow morning," Sammy affirmed.

Sammy and Abigail shook hands with Sergeant Bet and she drove off while they made their way up the small pathway that led to Uncle Goddy's gate.

They trotted along with their hands interlocked, "Should we ring the Insurance tonight?" Sammy asked.

"Yes, we should do that later," Abigail stated and then suddenly stepped into a pothole; flung away the bag she was holding and fell onto the ground.

Sammy quickly sprang to her aid, and lifted her from the ground, "Are you injured?"

"No, I don't think so." Abigail began dusting off dirt from her dress. "My skirt is wet."

"We'll sort it out when we get into the house," Sammy enjoined.

"I should have looked where I was going. I didn't see the pothole. I thought it was level ground."

"It was an accident. You know it's dark and it's really poorly lit on this pathway."

A few minutes later, Abigail made a slight grimacing sound.

"What's the matter? Are you sure that you didn't sustain any injury?"

"No, I'm fine," Abigail reiterated.

"So, what's the problem?" Sammy inquired.

"It seems I'm having some slight niggling tummy pain," she replied.

Abigail hadn't seen her period lately and did a home pregnancy test shortly before they left and it returned positive. It also indicated that she could be six weeks pregnant. She hadn't told her husband because she wanted to broach it after his father's burial. She is worried if there was any correlation of her sudden abdominal pain to the incident that they had experienced today. She thought that the best action is to dismiss that line of thought for now and then she shrugged.

"Why did you shrug?" Sammy asked her. "Has it anything to do with the tummy pain you've got?"

Abigail knew that she had to remain calm in order not to worsen her husband's alarmed state of mind.

"Nothing major," Abigail responded. "Let's keep going."

Sammy did as he was told, and they marched on.

As they were approaching the red letterbox, which stood as if on sentry duty for the gate, "I'm wondering which of the guards is on duty," Sammy said. "Uncle Goddy hires and fires at random."

"That would be necessary if one takes into consideration how dubious and ill-minded the so-called security guards could be," Abigail commented.

"You're absolutely correct. In fact, Uncle Goddy told me about a month ago that the most recent two he sacked were acting as insiders in a plot to have his house burgled and his wife's precious jewels carted away. However, luck ran out on them when one of his home help got wind of it and divulged the secret to another home help who then informed his wife."

Abigail shook her head, "He did well to have sacked them. It served them well."

Uncle Goddy's house is situated at the leafy end of Montana Park and was aptly named the Prince's Pavilion. It is a modern two-storey mansion which is befitting the calibre of a person like Uncle Goddy, who owns a private security company which has guards that patrol most streets in the city. His security guards have kept the hoodlums at bay from attacking him. Although that hasn't been without him working very hard at it.

The building would have to be perhaps only ten feet wide at the front, but it stretches some twenty feet back. It is beautifully oblong in shape. It's roof has extensions resembling a parked aeroplane sitting at an aerodrome. It has many rooms each serving different functions: two for study, four as bedrooms with en-suites, a large entertainment room, a dressing room and large garden in front with several Westringia Smokie garden vogue trees. It also has two isolated boy quarters on each side where the guards sleep. It is decorated with sliding windows from the ground to the top floor and is adorned with creamy coloured tiles on its brick walls and polished interior.

The mansion towers behind well-fortified iron gates, flanked by two sets of Juniperus Skyrocket tall trees crowned in grey, dancing gently in the wind.

Immediately Sammy and Abigail got closer to the gate, a security light came on. As Sammy was about to knock at the gate, it began to open as if it were remotely controlled.

A short while later, a stockily built, tall middle-aged male began to walk towards the gate from the east end of the compound, and shortly thereafter another shorter and younger man from the other end approached them. Both had their guns by their sides.

Both had been briefed about Sammy's arrival so they approached the gate with relaxed gaits

"How are you Sammy?" the older security guard asked.

"We're fine Jimmy," Sammy replied.

Jimmy is the oldest and longest serving employee of Uncle Goddy's. He's in his mid-50s and has been with Uncle Goddy for five years. He has a daughter in her late 20s who's living with his estranged wife in KwaZulu-Natal. His marriage failed some two years before he got employment with Uncle Goddy. The legal fees that he incurred from his separation left him a pauper and a recluse. He became so socially withdrawn that he could be taciturn whenever he attended any social gathering. He is, however, very reliable, business minded and trustworthy according to Uncle Goddy.

"How was your trip?"

"It was okay," Sammy lied.

At that point Jimmy looked in the direction of the junior guard, "Nathaniel, go back to your duty post," he commanded.

"Yes, Sir," Nathaniel replied and turned back.

Jimmy also turned around and headed back to his own duty post. He readjusted his gun which he had momentarily uncocked in case he had any surprises from the visitors. As he walked back, he appeared younger than his stated age of 55, in his load bearing vest which was worn on top of a pair of khaki trousers, and a short sleeved vest.

Suddenly Jimmy turned around, "Did somebody drop you people?" he asked.

"Yeah, you're correct," Sammy replied. Without waiting for the next question, "We had a mishap and our car is with the repairers."

"Hope it wasn't too badly damaged?" Jimmy asked in his thick Zulu accent.

"No, it wasn't," Sammy lied again.

Jimmy then trotted away.

Sammy didn't want to divulge the details of their ordeal to the security guards. Uncle Goddy wouldn't approve of it. Uncle Goddy had always warned him about his security guards, and often advised him to treat them with caution. Some of them, according to him, will often collude with armed robbers in the sense that they'll gather and release some vital internal sources of information and then receive payment for selling such information, or request to receive some share of the proceeds of the successful robbery.

Sammy and Abigail proceeded to the front of the building and the security guards disappeared from their view as they retreated to their duty posts.

As they approached the building, they saw Uncle Goddy who was already standing on his steps waiting for them. It seems the security light that had come on got his attention and he then came out to make sure it was Sammy and Abigail who were arriving into his compound.

He had been expecting them for over five hours. And knowing what South Africa is, he had become panic-stricken and worried that they had run into some problem. So, when he saw them now, he leapt into the air with joy.

With a wobbly gait he moved as fast as his bad hips and weak knees could carry him to them. "How are you Sammy?" he inquired as he hugged him then quickly turned to Abigail and hugged her too. He was initially undecided who to embrace first but then decided to start with his nephew.

Sammy and Abigail each embraced him individually. "How are you Uncle and Auntie Chelsea?" they asked.

"We're okay," he replied. "Chelsea has dozed off."

"Is she all right?" Abigail quizzed.

"She is okay apart from her usual tummy pain," he replied, then he immediately looked around and beyond them towards the gate, "Where's your car?"

"We had some problems on the way and had to leave it with the repairer," Sammy responded.

"Did it break down?"

"Not exactly," Sammy stopped, began to dig his right foot into the ground. "It was more than that."

When Sammy was a child, he used to dig into the ground with his right foot when he was in strife. Recognising Sammy's demeanour, Uncle Goddy wasn't relaxed anymore. "Let's get inside," he commanded them.

As they sauntered into the lounge room, Chelsea, Uncle Goddy's wife, rushed out to greet them, "I heard that your car broke down on the road, am I right?"

Abigail decided to respond, having observed that Sammy was still ill-at-ease, "We were chased but we survived it."

Uncle Goddy's mouth opened, shut and gaped again before it was finally closed. He shook his head and sank into a nearby lounge.

Geraldine, Sammy's mother who had rushed out from her room into the lounge room immediately dropped her big weight onto a wooden chair.

The rest of the family; Sammy's sister, Nancy, his brother Michael, and his wife, Agnes, as well as their Uncle Goddy's house help Tiny, all came into the lounge room to hear Sammy and Abigail's car hijack story.

Sammy slowly began to explain to them how they observed that they were being followed from the Flybuy Petrol Station at Kempton Park by hijackers.

Uncle Goddy shifted in his seat, "You called me when you were at the Petrol Station, am I not right?" he asked Sammy.

"You're right. Our ordeal started shortly after then."

He then went on to describe how Abigail alerted the Police who eventfully rescued them shortly after the hijackers had shot bullets that hit their car and were threatening to put bullets through their heads.

There was a deafening silence in the room apart from the slight noise from the television. Nobody spoke for some five minutes. They were all dumbfounded.

Tears began to run down Geraldine's face, Sammy's mum. She then burst into loud crying, "So I would've been burying both my husband and my son now."

She continued to shed tears inconsolably. Uncle Goddy reached out to her, "Ok, stop crying. They are here, alive and well." She didn't respond and continued weeping. He grabbed her arm, "Let's go to your room." He and Chelsea then led her into her room. Chelsea stayed with Geraldine and Uncle Goddy came back to the lounge room.

Sammy and Abigail also wandered into Geraldine's room and a short while later, Abigail came out and re-joined the others while Sammy stayed with her.

"We're lucky that there's no car hijacking in Australia," Michael commented.

"What'll happen now?" Uncle Goddy enquired.

"We'll attend the Police station tomorrow to make statements and then take our car to the garage if they have finished their forensic examination on it," Abigail responded.

"Did they do a lot of damage to the car?" Michael inquired.

"We're not sure yet," Abigail commented. "By our assessment, the bullet went through the petrol tank and that caused our car to roll."

Abigail tapped Tiny, "Please go to the gate, ask Jimmy, the security guard to give you the bag that I left at the gate. Take it into our room."

Tiny was glowing with happiness. She was thrilled that her favourite Uncle and his wife had arrived. She was however sad that they had had some mishap on their way. She hoped that things would work out well for them.

"Sure," Tiny responded and dashed out of the lounge room.

Some minutes later Uncle Goddy began to yawn and he stood up, stretching his arms and legs. "I'm retiring to bed," he announced. "I hope everybody knows where their rooms are?"

"Yes," they answered. "We'll be going to bed too."

Michael and Agnes walked to their room, whereas Abigail went to Geraldine's room and from there she and Sammy proceeded to theirs.

Chapter 5

Pretoria City Streets
Pretoria
South Africa
April 15, 1986, Tuesday

As Sammy and Abigail stepped out from their room which was adjacent to Michael's, Uncle Goddy was already sitting in the lounge room, sipping a cup of hot coffee which was his usual morning habit. He looked up and focused his gaze on them, "You two look gorgeous, indeed like a perfect match made in Heaven, I must say," he smiled.

"Thanks," Sammy and Abigail replied.

"Don't you want to sit down and have bites or two before heading off?" he asked them.

Abigail looked at the clock on the wall. "It's too early for us to eat," she replied.

"8.00 am is the perfect time for my morning coffee," Uncle Goddy chipped in.

"We will eat on our way back," Sammy suggested.

"That's okay, I've advised Pascal to drive you people to and from the Police Station. He'll also take you both to any other place that you would want to."

Pascal has been acting like the chauffeur for everybody in the house.

He was born and raised in Pretoria. He knows where the bad boys are and will dodge them. Uncle Goddy trusts him very much.

Turning to Pascal, "Make sure you avoid the car snatching route," Uncle Goddy advised.

"Sure, got to do so," Pascal replied in his thick Xhosa-rich dialect.

"Thank you, Uncle" Sammy chipped in.

"My pleasure."

Abigail quietly tapped Sammy on the elbow to remind him of something.

"Yeah, Uncle, what have the elders decided about my dad's burial date?" Sammy asked.

"They suggested that it should take place this Wednesday—that is the 16th."

Sammy lowered himself slowly to a chair next to Uncle Goddy, "Will there be enough time for preparation?" he asked.

"Most of the preparations have already been taken care of, dear." Looking up at Sammy, Uncle Goddy went on, "You know that it's our culture that burial must occur within a week or so after death."

Sammy lowered his face and nodded in acceptance. As he looked up, Michael and Geraldine walked into the room.

"It's better that we get it sorted out soon," Michael contributed. "Dad had requested some time ago for an early burial when he died."

Geraldine took a deep breath and sighed, "Michael is right; your father's wish was for an early burial. His desire was to limit the length of our moaning and crying." Her eyes became fuzzy with tears and she began to wail.

Sammy slowly stood up and moved over to Geraldine and to put his arm across her shoulders, "Stop crying Mama," he muttered.

Geraldine looked across the wall at the clock, "Oh my God, it's almost 9, and please, you two should get going."

Sammy and Abigail looked at each, then rose and walked out slowly out of the room.

They stepped out onto the veranda and then into the open space of the compound.

A cold breeze immediately hit Abigail's nostrils. "It's cold and wet this morning," she muttered.

"Yeah, you're damn right," Sammy confirmed.

The sky was dusky and dull. It was still drizzling, and the cool breeze was biting. It was like a sharp knife with a pointed edge. It certainly did penetrate Sammy's heart and he doubled up, as if he had been struck by a bullet. It exacerbated his sadness.

"What's wrong darling?" Abigail questioned.

"Just felt a chilling sensation in my heart," Sammy volunteered.

Reaching for his arm, Abigail egged him on, and they both rushed into the Mercedes car which was already steaming in wait for them.

"How are you two?" Pascal asked.

"We're fine," Sammy replied. Abigail nodded in acceptance of Sammy's response.

"Ah, it feels cosy inside here," Abigail was exhilarated. "Thanks for warming the car for us."

"You're welcome," Pascal replied. "I understand that you're going to the Pretoria City Old Police Station?"

"Yeah, you're correct," Sammy replied.

As the car was nudging through the gate, "I'd like us to go along the highway, or do you prefer through the city streets?" he asked.

"We prefer the City streets," Abigail replied. She had the premonition that they could suffer another hijacking experience.

Pascal slowed the car down momentarily as if weighing up the options he had given them. He nodded and commented, "Let's avoid the highway although it would appear to be safer."

Abigail cast a glance at her husband as if asking for his opinion. "What do you think?" she blurted out.

"You already have premonitions about the highway, and it seems to signify hijacking to you, so let's go through the City streets."

Abigail dropped her head in acquiescence, and they drove off.

Looking at them through the rear mirror, "It's a horrifying experience you people went through yesterday." Pascal commented.

"It's unbelievable," Sammy responded.

"You people were lucky to have survived it. Many won't."

"We know," Sammy replied brashly. He wasn't in the mood for long chats and would have to shut Pascal up.

Pascal seemed to have caught the joke. He quickly turned around and looked at Sammy and mumbled, "Sorry."

"It isn't your fault," Sammy replied and lowered his face.

Abigail looked at Sammy; his once adorable face now appeared gaunt and wrinkled with sadness. He managed to smile at her. Although he did that, she could see that it was hollow and was a façade that he had donned only as a mask to protect himself from receiving further probing questions. She reached out to him, and put her head on his right shoulder. "I love you," she promised.

Sammy gently put his right hand on Abigail's head which was resting on his shoulder. In a very small voice, he began to soliloquize; "I'm deeply sad and depressed. Sadness has eroded my bones and penetrated deep into my inner body. It flows in my blood through my veins and my arteries and has deadened my soul." He paused, lifted her head and looked into her eyes. Her eyes appeared grave and more penetrating than ever.

He returned to his original position and continued, "It is lethal to my spirit. It has poisoned and maimed every good emotion that I develop. It's like a cancer to my body. Chemo and radiotherapy won't rescue me. I'm not allowed to enjoy any break. It's a huge mist and dark cloud over me which have subdued me immeasurably. No matter how bright or sunny a day may be, I'm doomed. I can't see it and can't feel. My ears don't hear birds' songs anymore neither do my nostrils perceive the scents of flowers." He took a deep breath and continued, "Except when I remember that I've got a lovely wife in you."

Abigail stroked Sammy's arm, "It's okay Sammy, and all will be well, I promise," she said reassuringly.

Abigail had just finished speaking, when the car suddenly shook and came to an abrupt halt.

"Waooh, what's going on?" Sammy exclaimed as he was jarred back into reality.

"It seems he is drunk," Abigail stated as she observed a fellow crossing the road with a waddling gait.

"Sorry, I had to stop suddenly in order to avoid hitting him," Pascal explained.

"That's understandable," Sammy replied.

They were in the middle of Hill Street where there were malfunctioning traffic lights.

"This street is a beehive of activities now, whereas it was a ghost land last night when we drove through it," Abigail voiced.

Every house in the street had a unique structure and appearance. None seemed identical, either in architectural design or in colour to each other. Rather, some had pitched roofs, some zinc; some were only a single storey, some two and others three. They appeared as a disjointed set of teeth. The street had changed so much since Abigail went through it.

Just at the end of Hill Street, Sammy peered around as they were about to negotiate a turn into the main street, "How are we proceeding to the Police Station?" he asked.

"Given that you people don't want us to drive down the highways; we'll drive through the city which will see us go through Loftus Versfeld Rugby Stadium road, R4 Mainway, and R5 City link which will lead us into Klapperkop Nature Reserve main road where the Police Station is located. It's gonna be a long drive because of the traffic."

Sammy looked at Abigail only to enquire if she has had a change of mind as regards the route they should take.

Abigail gazed back at Sammy, "Let's go ahead through the route that you've outlined."

It wasn't long before they entered the Loftus Versfeld Rugby Stadium road that they were caught up in a traffic hold.

There were a lot of cars, each trailing one another, bumper to bumper, hooting and belching fumes. The traffic wound down the road like a great python, tyres often screeching and hissing on the wet road. They were starting and stopping incessantly, and the cars were bouncing down the road like green and brown frogs hopping into the lake.

As their car moved at a snail's pace trailing a blue Honda Civic which was driven by a lady, Abigail noticed that the lady's window was wound down, probably to allow the air in. And behind them was a motorcycle which was ridden by a thickly bearded, unshaven, unkempt, rough looking middle-aged man. He was wearing a short-sleeved shirt with a dark sleeveless jacket. He had thick dark glasses which covered his eyes. He wore a hat with the tip pointing backwards. He had no helmet and had tattoos on his exposed arms. The cyclist stopped each time they stopped, and rode off when they jerked forward. Abigail was getting concerned about the cyclist and was about to point that out to Sammy and Pascal when he immediately rode past them and pulled up by the side of the Honda Civic car. He stopped briefly and dipping his right hand into the side of his jacket, he pulled out something that looked like a short gun and placed it on the open window of the lady's car pointing it at her neck. He muttered something with a soft voice and the lady nodded quickly and immediately handed her handbag to him and he quickly rode off.

"Did you see what just happened?" Pascal asked.

"It's horrible that bags could be snatched in a traffic jam within seconds," Sammy commented.

Abigail felt sick in the pit of her stomach, she had headache, her heart began to pound and she was perspiring with trepidation, "We're lucky that our windows were wound up and not down otherwise he would have robbed us."

"The lady is very unlucky and partly to be blamed for winding her window down. That's an invitation to the armed bandits to attack." Pascal said and shook his head.

As they were discussing the incident, they observed the lady leave the trail of traffic and park her car on the side of the road, then got out.

Pascal drove beyond the lady's car and parked theirs. They all got out to render some help to her. Other cars passed by as if they were oblivious of her and her predicament.

As they got close to her, Sammy began the introductions. "Hello, my name is Sammy," he said. He pointed to his left, "This is Abigail and she's my wife." He turned to his right, "This is Pascal, our driver," and then extended a hand to shake hers.

The lady was a Caucasian of average height. She looked to be in her late 30s. She had dishevelled blonde frizzy hair, some falling into her mouth under the slight wind. She appeared as white as a ghost, her arms and lips were trembling, and her teeth were clattering as if she had caught a cold, although the weather had become warmer. Her legs were quivering and appeared to be about to give way under her. She struggled to mumble out words.

They felt pity for the lady.

She extended her hand to meet Sammy's. The vibrations of her hand made Sammy feel like he was going to be electrocuted.

"I'm Beckie O'Gradey," she responded. Then she turned to the other two, and with a quavering voice, asked, "How are you Abigail and Mr Pascal."

The duo returned the pleasantry.

"Do you need any help?" Sammy asked politely.

The lady took a deep breath, "Yeah, I would have wanted to alert the police and my husband."

"Have you done so?" Sammy asked.

"No."

"Why?"

"My cell phone was in the bag that the thief snatched."

Immediately, Abigail pulled her phone out of her purse and gave it to the lady to make the phone calls.

"Hello Darling, I've been robbed at gun point," Beckie told her husband.

"Where're you?" her husband questioned.

"In a traffic jam in the middle of Loftus Versfeld Rugby Stadium road," Beckie replied.

"Whose phone are you calling from?"

"Passers-by who saw what happened and stopped to help me,"

"Okay, what a hell of a day," her husband ejaculated. "Do you still have your car with you?"

Beckie was appearing more flustered. "Yes, I do."

"What did they take?"

"My bag," she replied and began to wail.

"Stop crying darling. Please drive to the Pretoria City Old Police Station. I'll meet you there soon."

In between her sobs, Beckie replied, "Okay, I'll do so."

She gave the phone back to Abigail. "Thanks very much."

As Abigail was receiving her phone back from Beckie, two other drivers pulled over close to Beckie's car.

The first, a middle-aged black man, approached Beckie and handed a piece of paper to her. "It's got the motor cyclist's plate number."

"Thanks immensely," Beckie replied.

"I can't vouch that it's accurate, but it could however give the police a lead," the man said.

"It'll certainly help," Beckie replied.

"I've got to go," the man announced and jumped into his car and drove off.

As the first person was leaving, the second person who was a lady approached Beckie and introduced herself. "I'm Lucy. I've got an important piece of evidence for you."

Beckie was bewildered and looked at her with her mouth ajar.

Lucy brought out her cell phone and flicked through the pictures and pointed to one, "Look, I took a picture of the man because I sensed that he was about to rob somebody, so I was prepared for it."

"Did you take any as he was robbing me?" Beckie inquired.

"Sure, I did," Lucy replied.

Joining in the discussion, Sammy and Abigail exclaimed, "That's amazing and good of you."

"I'm grateful for this piece of evidence," Beckie chipped in. "Are you happy to attend the Police Station with me?"

"Sure, I'm happy to do so. These hoodlums should be caught and dealt with," Lucy reassured her.

"Let's head off to the Police Station before the thief makes it too far," Sammy stated.

"You're absolutely right Sir," Lucy confirmed.

They all began to retreat to their respective cars.

Sammy tapped Abigail, "I think I should drive that lady's car for her, I don't think that she's in a frame of mind to drive."

Abigail nodded, "Please, can you ask her first if she needs that type of help."

Sammy went across to the lady and tapped on her window as she was still fiddling with the car key trying to start the engine, "My wife asked if you would want me to drive you to the Police Station. We're going there ourselves."

The lady looked at Sammy and was speechless for some seconds. "I can't believe that you and your wife could be this helpful." She took a deep breath. "It'll be a great relief if you could drive me as I'm in a shattered state of mind and quite sure that I'll struggle to move this car."

Abigail approached them at that instant, "Darl, I'll join Pascal and we'll follow."

Sammy jumped into the lady's car and drove, and Abigail and Pascal followed them behind.

Chapter 6

Pretoria City Old Police Station
Klapperkop Nature Reserve road
Pretoria, South Africa
April 15, 1986, Tuesday

Making it to the Police Station beyond the bag snatching point was relatively hitch-free and not as hectic and traumatising for Sammy and Abigail as it had been for them driving from Hill Street. The traffic jam had also cleared reasonably to the extent that both Abigail and Sammy were able to reach the Police Station before their appointment time of 11.00 am.

Immediately Sammy drove Beckie into the Police Station he looked around and went straight to the Visitor's Car Park, "Hope you can take care of yourself from now on?" he asked Beckie.

"Sure, I can." She looked around and noted her husband's car at the end of the car park. "My husband is over there."

As Sammy was opening the door, he advised Beckie, "I need to get off to meet my wife so that we can get into the station for our appointment."

Beckie sluggishly lifted her legs, one after the other as if they weighed several tonnes of kilos and then got out of her car and began to walk towards her husband, knowing that he would be waiting for her. After taking a few steps, she remembered that she did not actually thank Sammy. The shock and sadness of the bag snatching had clouded her memory and she couldn't focus or think straight. She quickly turned around and saw Sammy a distance away and then screamed with the little energy left in her, "I'm very grateful for the help you've rendered to me."

She wasn't sure that Sammy would hear, but surprisingly he turned around and waved at her. He then walked into the corridor of the Police Station where Abigail was already waiting for him.

As he was stepping onto the front stairs of the corridor, he hit the edge of the stair which had broken but had not been repaired. It dawned on him that this police building was being neglected.

The Pretoria City old Police Station sits conspicuously at the intersection of Klapperkop Nature Reserve Road and Great Southern Highway overlooking the Freedom Park Game Reserve. The building is a low-set, U shaped, single storey, made of a mixture of timbers on its east end and concrete on the west wing. It's painted in yellow and could do with some repainting because the coating on its walls has peeled off in most areas. It has obviously not received much attention by way of renovations or refurbishment since it was built in 1903; thanks to the corrupt politicians and managers who have continuously embezzled funds ear-marked for it.

The Police Station has Police Staff Quarters at its rear and administrative buildings in the front. The former houses Police personnel, their vehicles and their personal effects, whereas the latter have temporary holding cells, interview and interrogation rooms.

The main administrative office is a simple rectangular room 16 feet by 16 feet separated from two cells.

"Darling, you almost hit the ground," Abigail observed.

"Yeah, I almost hit the floor but was able to avoid it."

Abigail shook her head in disbelief, "I wonder why it is that nobody has noticed this crack?"

"Or noticed it, but hasn't cared to repair it," Sammy chipped in.

He put his arm around Abigail and they began to walk towards the main administrative offices.

Before entering the main building, he looked up at the entrance and noticed a -Statement of Significance- which was written in bold:

"The Pretoria City Old Police Station has high historical and social significance to the City and the Council for its associations in 1840 when the first permanent White inhabitants arrived in Pretoria and 1855 when the City became officially recognised."

He pointed it out to Abigail, "Darling, do you comprehend this Statement of Significance?" he asked.

"The Statement probably depicts the significant and pivotal role which the Police Station played in Pretoria City Council's law enforcement history."

"Hello Sammy and Abigail, how have you guys been?" Constable Kagiso asked.

They looked in his direction and saw him standing in front of them.

"We're fine," Sammy replied. Abigail nodded in confirmation of her husband's assertion.

"I guess you would be looking for Sergeant Bet," Constable Kagiso inquired.

"Is she the person who should be interviewing us?" Sammy replied.

"I think she is the right person to see as she'll direct you to the CID officer who is in charge of your case."

"Ok, so what should we do now?"

Constable Kagiso pointed them to the visitors' chairs that were at the end of room, "Please sit there. The clerical officers will take some details from you while I go and find her for you people."

Sammy and Abigail quickly made themselves comfortable on a wooden set of chairs beside the entrance door. As they did, Constable Kagiso disappeared into the opposite hallway.

A young lady in her early 30s who wore what looked like bifocal lenses leaned across the counter and called out "Hello, can you please come forward."

As they were making their way to the front of the counter to give their details, the young girls quickly abandoned them, sprang out and dashed out very fast to the far end of building from where a loud noise could be heard.

In that instance, Sammy and Abigail noticed that the commotion was significant, and it was coming from the far end of the building where the clerical officers had dashed off to.

The chaotic noise could be likened to a pre-school or kindergarten classroom on the first day of school when the teacher has either turned up late or has not turned up at all. Ordinarily, Abigail's sight is not very reliable and on this day when she has been dazzled by several events, she could not focus to ascertain the cause of the rowdiness. She looked very hard but could not comprehend what the problem was.

Sammy also looked and looked but saw little. He shook his head. "What's happening?"

"Only heaven knows." Abigail muttered and looked up to the sky and then back to Sammy.

As Sammy and Abigail were eyeing each other, trying to decipher the cause of the noise, the noise seemed to be coming into the building.

Abigail felt like running away, but the reassuring look on the face of her husband kept her standing. She clung to Sammy tightly as if she was being drowned.

Sammy extricated himself from the clutches of his wife. "Sit down Darling," he urged her. "I need to know what's going on here."

He then walked to a nearby window and peered through.

"Darling, it's a large crowd of people." He poked his head through the window protectors. "It seems the crowd is intending to lynch somebody."

At that instance, Abigail sprang to her feet and joined Sammy. "What do you think is happening?"

Sammy spotted Pascal and yelled out at him and the latter came to come to the window. "What's happening?"

"Do you recall the motor cyclist who snatched the lady's handbag at gun point? He has been caught." He paused. "It seems that the people were about to put a tyre on his neck to set him alight when the Police appeared."

"And what next ...?" Abigail quizzed.

Pascal began to explain the next set of events even before Abigail finished her sentence. "The police stopped the mob carrying out their intention."

"The police obviously have saved the man," Sammy chipped in.

"I won't say so," Pascal commented. "The police and the lynching mobs are wrestling to see which side will have the upper hand."

"Which side has the upper hand?" Sammy asked.

"It seems like the police requested back-up and they used tear gas to free the man from the people."

"Is that why they are all approaching the Police Station now?" Abigail queried.

"Yeah, it seems so."

It was not long before the crowd started streaming into the Police Station.

The first to enter was the cyclist in handcuffs surrounded by four heavily armed police officers. Following them was Beckie and a man beside her.

Beckie walked in measured steps as if she was still in shock. She quickly recognised Abigail and Sammy and came and sat beside them.

As she sat down, the man who came in with her sat beside her. "Darling, this is the couple who helped me after the attack."

The man extended his hand to Sammy, "I am Tim."

"He's my husband, just to complete the introduction. I guess you've realised by now."

"Of course, we figured it out," Abigail commented with a smile. "So, he was eventually caught?"

"Yeah, nemesis has caught up with him today," Beckie responded. "He didn't know that my husband was just a stone's throw away when he robbed me."

Abigail and Sammy seemed a bit flabbergasted. "What did your husband do to apprehend him?" Abigail asked.

Tim stepped into the discussion and went on, “When I heard of the robbery, I mobilised the local vigilante as we were the only two of us on patrol.” He shook his head and continued. “Little did I know that my wife was the victim.”

“So, what happened thereafter?” Sammy quizzed him.

“Usually, the vigilante will carry out what is described as necklacing.” He stopped as he heard his wife’s name being called. “They want you to attend the front counter for collection of basic information about you.” He told his wife. “Darling, go ahead. I’ll be with you for the actual interview.”

He relaxed back with Sammy and Abigail to continue with his story.

“So what’s necklacing?” Abigail queried.

“Necklacing is actually a form of extrajudicial summary killing or execution, if you may, whereby torture is carried out by placing a rubber tyre filled with petrol around an alleged robber’s neck and setting it on fire. The person will have a miserable death. He or she will be literally roasted to death. The death usually occurs within 20 – 30 minutes after the tyre has been lit up.”

Sammy wished that it was done to this man, to deter others from that type of life style. “Why was it not done to this man?”

“The man was lucky, because my collagues had already called for back-up before the vigilantes could get their act together.” Tim explained further.

At this time, the clerical officer walked back to her chair and beckoned Sammy and Abigail to come over to her to release their details.

“Darling, you can go and give them the details,” Sammy encouraged his wife.

The two men continued their discussion. “Were the vigilante armed?” Sammy asked.

“Some had locally made guns which would not have matched what the armed robber had.” Tim responded.

“So how did they apprehend the armed robber, given that his gun was smarter than theirs?”

"My colleague and I had engaged in gun battle till he had no pellets left and that's when the vigilante swarmed in on him."

As he was describing that, another man walked through a door just behind where Sammy and Tim sat.

He quickly sat beside Tim and shook hands with him. "This is one of the vigilante members."

"Thanks for introducing him," Sammy stated.

"I'm Marshall," the vigilante member told Sammy.

"I'm Sammy." They shook hands. "So, who're you people?"

"We're called a vigilante group because we have members who have volunteered their time. We believe that the law and its processes are inadequate to control crime successfully because of which it is blossoming. We're practically local men who are organised to suppress and punish crime outside the realms of official court rooms."

"So, you summarily execute a person or persons who you think have committed evil?"

"Sammy, it must be abundantly clear that the person or persons in question have robbed or killed an innocent person before we take him or her out."

Although Sammy was enjoying it, he wanted to gain more insight into how the vigilante group operated. "Is it fair to say that you people are self-appointed doers of justice?"

"If you want to address us like that, then that's okay." He paused. "All I know is that we try to keep the crime rate very low, or if possible, control it completely."

"Don't you think that the Court system does the same thing?"

Marshall chuckled, "I beg to defer."

As they were conversing, the cyclist was led across where the men were sitting, still in handcuffs.

"He appears extremely subdued now in comparison to his demeanour on the road," Sammy commented sizing the man up as he was led away into another cell.

As he looked up, he saw that his wife was coming back to him and at the same time, Sergeant Bet was approaching them from another angle of the building.

He welcomed Abigail and they waited for Sergeant Bet to get to them.

They also noted that Beckie had re-joined her husband.

"Can we go to my office?" Sergeant Bet asked Sammy and Abigail.

"We'll certainly meet again," Sammy told Tim and Beckie as the duo stood up and followed Sergeant Bet.

"Sure, we will," Tim replied.

As they were all walking to Sergeant Bet's room, they narrated to Sergeant Bet the events that they had witnessed that day.

"Do you know that this cyclist was among the group of robbers who attacked you people yesterday?" Sergeant Bet announced to them in the hallway.

In profound consternation, "How did you know?" Abigail asked.

"We've had records coming which have confirmed it," she replied.

"Records from where?" asked Sammy.

"Information from insiders – such as undercover police and other intelligent sources."

"Do you think that he'll confess to confirm it?" Abigail questioned.

"In due course, he will."

At that time, they walked into her office. "Please make yourselves comfortable."

They both sat on the lounge chair which was adjacent to the door.

"Can I offer you anything? We've got coffee and water."

"You can give me water, thank you," Sammy stated.

"Mrs Petters, what about you?"

"Thanks, water will be okay for me also."

She brought the water, and as they were drinking, she discussed the case and the progress they had made so far.

"The driver confessed to us and gave important clues which we'll be following up on shortly.

"Did the driver inform you that the motorcyclist was one of them?" Abigail asked.

"Yes, he did."

"What should we expect next, or what are we expected to do now?" Sammy enquired.

"The driver and his gang will be arraigned in court. Hopefully, we'll be able to extract the same level of confession from him."

"Given that he has already confessed now, and you've got it on tape, do you think he could change?" Abigail chipped in.

"Unlikely, although it could still be possible."

"After the Court case, what will happen next?" Sammy quizzed her.

"The Court will likely direct that you to be paid some money from the Victims Compensation Scheme money."

"Where's our car?" Sammy enquired.

"We dropped it back to the garage this morning. The Forensic team finished with it last night, knowing that you'll not be able to drive to the garage, so we towed it to the Moonlight Crash Repairs for you people."

"Thanks, we'll go to the garage, review it and then we'll contact the Insurance company for a loan car."

They shook hands and Sergeant Bet ushered them out the door.

On exiting out from Sergeant Bet's office, Sammy located Pascal having a conversation with a vigilante member. "Hey Pascal, we're done for now, can you please take us back home?" Sammy asked him.

"Sure, let's get going," he announced in high spirits. Turning to his companion, he said, "I'm keen on becoming a member. We shall talk in detail in future."

"You've got my mobile number, contact me whenever you want," the member replied and waved at him.

Immediately they reached the park where their car was, and were about to enter, Abigail's steps began to wobble. "What's wrong?" Sammy asked as he rushed to support her.

"Take me to a clinic or a hospital now," she babbled.

Chapter 7

Streets of City Centre
To Life Matters Best Hospital
No 40 Georgina Avenue
Groenkloof 0281, Pretoria
South Africa
April 15, 1986, Tuesday, 2.00 pm

Upon uttering those words Abigail crumpled down. Half of her was inside and the other half outside the car. Her left leg was trapped inside and the right outside, as she was attempting to step into the car when she became floppy.

Noticing the unfolding crisis, Pascal rushed to help Sammy, "Let's get her into the car," Sammy commanded.

They both helped Abigail into the car. Pascal pulled open the driver's door and jumped in behind the steering wheel, whereas Sammy squeezed himself beside Abigail in the back seat trying as much as possible not to inconvenience her.

Sammy shook her, "Darling, are you all right?" he sang out. His own heart was pounding. He felt beads of perspiration falling down his face and dimming his vision. Goose flesh was palpable all over him. She had never been this ill to his knowledge. Whatever the cause of her illness, he resolved to wade through it with her. She is his sunshine and without her, the sun will never rise again.

Abigail was breathing heavily. She was not responding but her eyes were flickering. "I don't feel well," she whispered. "Take me to a hospital please."

Sammy looked at Pascal, and Pascal cast a glance back at him. "I'm not sure what we should do," Pascal announced with a quivering voice.

"Let's hit the road please," Sammy commanded.

Pascal revved the engine, but was undecided as to where to head to, so he stopped the car. He however kept the engine on so to cool the inside of the car for Abigail and Sammy. He then grabbed his mobile phone and stepped out of the car and began to dial some numbers.

At that instant, having witnessed what was happening from the window of her office, Sergeant Bet came rushing out. "What's going on, guys?"

Before Sammy could respond, she continued, "It seems your wife is very ill?"

With a deep breath, Sammy looking at her through the window which he had wound down responded, "Yeah, you're right."

"Let's call the ambulance," she volunteered, and then rushed back into her office to make some phone calls.

While Sergeant Bet was conversing with Sammy, Pascal rang Uncle Goddy.

"Abigail has collapsed Sir."

"What happened?" Uncle Goddy enquired.

"I'm not sure exactly. She and Sammy came out from Sergeant Bet's officer and they were about to enter the car when she reported feeling wobbly on her legs ..."

Uncle Goddy interrupted him, "Who's Sergeant Bet?"

"That's the Police Officer in charge of their case."

Uncle Goddy was not sure what he was hearing, "She was not being detained by any Police Officer, am I right?"

Pascal quickly understood that Uncle Goody wanted to ascertain that she didn't collapse because she feared that she would be detained. "We were about to head home when she collapsed."

"Where's she now?" Uncle Goddy questioned.

"She's lying inside the car."

"Where's Sammy?"

"He's with her in the car," Pascal clarified.

"What's the plan?" He paused and before Pascal could reply, "Do you people intend calling the ambulance for her?"

"Sir, I'm not sure what the plan is," Pascal responded.

"Let me talk to Sammy."

Pascal walked back to the car and gave the phone to Sammy. "Uncle Goddy's on the line."

As he received the phone from Pascal, Sammy asked, "Is this phone on speaker?"

Pascal nodded, "So that we can all converse at the same time."

"Hello Uncle," Sammy greeted.

"Hello Sammy. I've heard that Abigail collapsed, am I right?"

"Yeah, not exactly, she felt weak and before she collapsed, I lowered her onto the back seat of the car."

"Do you know what's wrong with her?"

"She indicated that she has tummy pain and she's still pointing to her abdomen as the source of her problem."

"Ehh – m," Uncle Goddy became silent for some fractions of minutes. "Okay, she needs a good specialist gynaecologist hospital as soon as possible," he asserted.

"Like where, have you got a guide for us?" Sammy was concerned and worried.

"Sure. I think Sisters of Mary Hospital, springs to mind as the best place to take to her to."

"Where's the hospital and how do we locate it?" Sammy blurted out.

"Pascal knows the direction. It is a bit far from where you are now." He paused again. "Pascal has been there several times. He took me to that hospital when I had an infection in my hip. The doctors there saved me by giving me a hip replacement."

Pascal chipped in, "I know the route and the direction but the traffic jam through the City Centre might hamper us getting there on time."

"You're correct, I think Abigail is seriously ill and needs urgent medical attention."

As they were conversing, Sergeant Bet re-joined them, "The Ambulance is a bit tied up now. The quickest time for an ambulance arriving here is in another 45 minutes."

Sammy pointed to the speaker on the phone and relayed to Sergeant Bet, "My Uncle is on the phone."

"Hello Sir, I'm Sergeant Bet, I am looking after Sammy and Abigail's case," she paused.

"Hello Sergeant, I'm Goddy Petters, Sammy's big uncle." With a calm and commanding voice, he went on, "How can you help them transfer Abigail to Sisters of Mary Hospital which is at the outskirts of Pretoria?"

"Ambulance would've been the quickest and fastest mode of transport, but I'm afraid to inform you that we don't have any available right now."

"I've been on the phone for the past 10 minutes and that's the result of my conversation with Paramedics headquarters here in Pretoria."

"Okay, it seems we're in dire straits right now."

Sergeant Bet raised her eyebrows in frustration, "Sounds like that Sir."

As they were still deliberating, Sammy appraised Abigail from head to toe. Heaved a sigh and shook her. "How're you doing Darling?"

With a voice barely audible, Abigail responded, "I still have tummy pain."

"Is it getting worse?"

"Yeah, Darling."

"We'll soon be on the way." Sammy reassured her.

Abigail nodded. She has always had a placid and stable personality. It takes a lot to get her complaining, or angry or frazzled. She has a very high pain threshold. Sammy understands that when Abigail complains of pain she is not playing.

"Do you have any clue why you've got such pain?" Sammy pryed.

Abigail signalled that she needed to write as she was too weak to talk. Sammy produced a pen and paper. She wrote, "No menses."

As they were deliberating on what Abigail had written, they noticed a Police vehicle pull out from behind the building.

"Let's get going guys," Sergeant Bet announced as she hopped out of the vehicle briefly to issue instructions to all of them. "We're going to Sisters of Mary Hospital, am I right?"

"Yeah, Sergeant." Sammy replied.

"The driver knows the hospital. Our vehicle will lead the way and we'll clear the road for you people."

Sammy's face beamed up hope. "Thanks immensely Sergeant Bet."

Pascal was elated. "We'll follow you closely."

"She's an angel." Uncle Goddy exclaimed. "I'll contact the hospital now."

"Cheers and bye Uncle," Sammy uttered.

The Police van activated its sirens and Pascal followed behind. Off they went from the Police compound and headed to the main street.

Uncle Goddy rang Sammy back some minutes later and sought to know how Abigail was going.

"She still has the tummy pain but seems more stable."

"Are you on the way now?"

"We are indeed."

"How's the traffic affecting you people?"

"We're moving very fast, traversing the street, jumping traffic lights and skipping hold-ups with the help of the Police vehicle with its sirens."

"Sammy, I hope you're holding yourself together?" Uncle Goddy paused. "Abigail needs you."

"I'm doing so." Sammy replied. "Have you told my mum of what has happened?"

"Not really." Sammy heard him grind his teeth. "I guess I wanted to secure a solution or something that looks like it before breaking the news to her."

Sammy was getting concerned also about his mother. "What has she been doing since morning?" he asked.

"She's been resting. I'll be in touch with you soon."

"Thanks uncle."

"Keep an eye on that priceless jewel of ours." Uncle Goddy announced with a tone of finality.

"Sure, I'll do so." Sammy replied.

Sammy is sure that Uncle Goddy will be ringing Sisters of Mary Hospital right now. Uncle Goddy has had a great fatherly disposition towards him and his siblings even when their father was alive. He has always been a pillar of strength and support for all of them. He springs to action whenever they are in need and they call upon him. He is their source of courage and encouragement. Although he is well to do because he has worked very hard all through his life, he has remained very humble in his wealth. He treats everyone with great respect and more importantly, leads by example rather than by precepts only.

Sammy is grateful that they still have Uncle Goddy as he knows that he'll protect them.

"Did you see how that cyclist tried to overtake us?" Pascal asked.

The question jarred Sammy back to reality. "He was lucky that the Police vehicle didn't knock him down."

Pascal quickly glanced at the rear mirror and noticed that Sammy's head has dropped again.

He felt sorry for Sammy and wished he could do more for him. "She'll be fine," Pascal encouraged him.

"I hope so," Sammy replied and began admiring his sleeping angel again.

To Sammy, this is the scariest journey of his life. His fear has been made worse by the fact that he doesn't know if Abigail will make it to the hospital. He has observed that Abigail's eyes often roll up and down and at other times will remain perfectly shut. She isn't able to speak in sentences although often will make an effort to vocalise her symptoms. The best she has done so far is when she pointed to her tummy and reported, "It still hurts." After saying that, she faded off again and appeared as white as a ghost.

Abigail is not only attractive physically but has a perfect personality. She has beautiful long blonde hair, with perfectly set blue eyes. When she smiles her cheekbones appear like those of an angelic creature from a celestial planet. When she speaks, her adoring sing-song voice will attract you to her.

Above all these, she is very supportive and Sammy's best friend. She shows interest in Sammy's interests and does not hesitate to express and show her love for him. He describes her as his soul mate and companion.

"It's a sharp knife through my heart, to see her in this state," he soliloquised.

Pascal nodded. "All will be well."

Abigail was unable to communicate anything more to Sammy no matter how hard he probed throughout the trip to the hospital. He attributed her lack of communication to her abdominal pain which had led her to variable low level of consciousness.

Sammy often wondered if Abigail would ever make it to the hospital alive. She often grimaced and displayed flickering expressions of pain on her face, and at other times coiled up on Sammy's arm. Sammy often entertained a flickering thought that even if she made it to the hospital; she may not survive. He struggled and dismissed the thoughts when they intruded into his consciousness.

To him it was like an endless journey. Whenever he saw a hospital sign on the road, he hoped that would be the Sisters of Mary Hospital. His hopes were on several occasions dashed as their car would speed past the sign and carry on down the highway.

As they were driving, he heard Uncle Goddy converse with Pascal and enquired how they were going. Pascal told him that they would be inside the Sisters of Mary Hospital in 10 minutes.

As Pascal and Uncle Goddy were conversing, another vehicle overtook their Mercedes and at that time Pascal lost sight of the Police vehicle. He had neither Sergeant Bet's number nor that of her driver.

"Hello Sammy, do you have Sergeant Bet's mobile number?" Pascal asked.

He mumbled, "I do somewhere." He began to rummage in his pocket for the business card that Sergeant Bet gave them a night ago.

"If you can't find it then, I'll find a way and negotiate through the traffic so that we can still get to the hospital soon."

Sammy searched everywhere but couldn't find the card. "I think she actually gave the card to Abigail."

"Okay, let's keep going then," Pascal stated.

"How are you going to negotiate through the traffic jam and hold-ups?" Sammy asked.

"I'll switch on my hazard lights and that could force other cars off the road and away from ours, hopefully."

Sammy was delighted that Pascal came up with that idea as he wanted any trick that would shorten their trip. "I'm glad that you're quick thinking. I'll not want us to be caught in the traffic any longer than necessary."

Pascal did as he had stated and that helped them to move reasonably faster until they got to a traffic light.

"Do you want to run through the light?" Sammy asked.

"I don't think that the hazard lights alone will compel other vehicles to give way to us at the traffic light."

Sammy pondered. "I don't think it's safe to do so."

At that point they reached the traffic light.

"This is Groenkloof District traffic light. It's the last light before we branch into Georgina Drive where the hospital is located." Pascal commented.

"That's good." Sammy replied.

Turning his gaze to his wife again, he shook her gently, "Are you still with us, Darling?"

Abigail gave him thumps up. That brought a smile to his face.

As Sammy looked up, the Police vehicle was in the middle of the traffic light directing their Mercedes to follow them. "That's them, they realised that they'd lost us and came back searching for us."

"Sergeant Bet is a legend. She is too good." Pascal commended.

"You're absolutely correct," Sammy confirmed.

Pascal followed the Police vehicle and they ran through the red light and veered into Georgina Drive towards the Sisters of Mary Hospital.

Upon sighting the street sign which read Georgina Drive, Sammy felt joyous. He now began to feel more positive that his wife would survive and how she would be after the treatment.

Pascal glanced at Sammy through the mirror. "Sammy, just keep calm and collected. She will fine."

Sammy looked up at him, tears rolling down his face. He uttered no response.

Pascal noticed that the Police vehicle had gone beyond the hospital gate and made a U-turn. Sergeant Bet had also got out and had beckoned him to drive in.

"We've got another call out to attend. Wishing you the best," she waved at them and jumped back into their vehicle which then headed back to the City Centre.

Pascal continued and drove their Mercedes into the Sisters of Mary Hospital premises.

Chapter 8

Life Matters Best Hospital
No 40 Georgina Avenue
Groenkloof 0281, Pretoria
South Africa
April 15, 1986, Tuesday, 3.00 pm

As soon as the Mercedes negotiated beyond the gate, Sammy was astounded by how beautiful and rich the Sisters of Mary Hospital was. "It's magnificent," he exclaimed.

Pascal agreed. "It's the best within this area and their services are second to none."

The opulent 100-bed Life Matters Best Hospital is situated in a hilly, leafy suburb north-west of Pretoria, about five miles from its city centre. It used to be manned by the Sisters of Mary in early 2000 and was then known as the Sisters of Mary Hospital. The name change came about when the two founding Reverend Sisters were killed in a ghastly motor accident, and new owners were appointed by the government. While the name may have changed, the hospital still contends that the doctors and staff have continued to serve the community and its patients with unswerving dedication, embracing the values of commitment, compassion, competence and spiritual support.

A short distance from the entrance, a glowing signage reads

"The hospital has a worldwide reputation for the treatment of gynaecological and neurological problems in its specially equipped

theatres. The state-of-the-art facilities include six theatres specifically designated for gynaecological procedures and five theatres for neurological cases as well as a trauma centre with special resuscitation facilities. A large team of renowned specialists— 14 gynaecological, 12 neurological, and 10 medical doctors are available to patients in this world-class facility. We pride ourselves on our ability to deliver excellent healthcare and embrace the principles of dedication, empathy, excellence and empowerment."

Scanning around, "Where are you going to drop us?" Sammy asked.

"We're going straight to the Emergency Department."

As Pascal was approaching the Emergency Department, Sammy noticed that there were two nurses and two doctors standing at the entrance door. One of the nurses was holding a stretcher. One of the doctors was older; as were the two nurses; one looked older than the other. Sammy wasn't sure if they were waiting for them or not.

"Hello Mr Pascal, is that the patient in the back seat?" the old doctor enquired as Pascal brought the car to a halt. "We already have some information about her."

"Yeah, she is," Pascal affirmed.

I'm Dr Simon OsGood and my assistant is Dr Prince DoLittle. The head nurse is Sister Angelina and her assistant is Sister Kate.

Dr OsGood immediately began to check Abigail's response state. "Please bring the stretcher and let's get Mrs Petters onto it," he announced.

They all swiftly swung into action and within a second Abigail was already on the stretcher.

Within a fraction of a second, they were already wheeling Abigail into the Emergency Department.

The Emergency Department was a beehive of activities; there were about 10 cubicles each sectioned off with curtains. Machines were beeping everywhere, and people were trooping in and out in orderly fashion from one end of the building to the other like marching soldier ants making their way to and from their ant hills.

To help them navigate, an orderly was called in who directed other people out of their path as they wheeled Abigail to the designated cubicle.

Sammy was astonished at their level of organisation, professionalism, dedication and commitment. He was also very glad that they were super-efficient.

As they were walking through the Emergency Department, Dr OsGood quickly produced a piece of notepaper from the side pocket of his clinical coat. He looked at it and turned around. "Which of you is Sammy, Abigail's husband?" He asked looking at Sammy and Pascal who were behind him.

Sammy came forward. "It's me, Dr OsGood."

"How are you Sammy?"

"I'm better now that we're here." He took a breath. "And how are you Doc?"

"I'm great." Dr OsGood stopped briefly and continued. "From the look of things your wife is not well, so I'll surmise that you've been scared stiff if she'll make it into our hospital. Is that right?"

Sammy nodded.

"Mr Goddy Petters, I believe he's your uncle, rang and advised us that you were heading our way."

"He hinted to me that he would be doing that," Sammy responded.

"Let's take her to cubicle 10," Dr OsGood announced.

They did as he commanded and took Abigail to the far end of the Emergency room where cubicle 10 was.

Inside the cubicle, Dr OsGood turned his attention to Abigail. He tapped her gently on the shoulder. "Open your eyes for me."

Abigail opened her eyes.

"Do you know where you are?"

Abigail was too weak to give a response.

"Are you okay?" Dr OsGood asked.

She shook her head.

"Where's the problem?"

She pointed to her tummy.

"Do you have a problem anywhere else?" Dr OsGood inquired.

She shook her head again.

"I gather that you've not seen your period?"

She nodded.

"I see," Dr OsGood exclaimed. And then he reached for a portal Ultrasound machine adjacent to her bed and with it, he did a bedside scanning of Abigail's abdomen and pelvic area. He noted fluid collections in the abdomen and pouch of Douglas.

He shook his head. "Mrs Petters needs fluid immediately. I need a cannula and drip giving set."

Sister Angelina brought what he requested. Dr OsGood inserted the cannula and collected blood in tubes and handed them to Dr DoLittle.

"Sister Angelina please, set up a bag of normal saline 0.9% to go in at the fastest rate now."

Sister Angelina beckoned to Sister Kate to bring the trolley which had the fluid bag and they hooked it onto Abigail.

"After the bag of normal saline, what else should we set up?" Sister Angelina asked.

"You can connect another bag of normal saline."

"Sure, we'll do so."

Dr OsGood, then turned to his assistant, "Dr DoLittle, please ring the theatre and inform them that we have a lady who has acute abdomen; differentials include ectopic pregnancy and ruptured ovarian cyst. And will likely need exploratory laparotomy."

"Should I contact the surgical team also?" Dr DoLittle asked.

"Sorry, you're right, we need the surgeons. Please send the bloods to the laboratory. Please request for urgent grouping and cross-matching, BHCG and other relevant tests."

As attempts at resuscitating Abigail were afoot, Sister Angelina hooked her up onto the monitors.

As he finished giving directions to his junior, Dr OsGood looked at the monitor.

"She's got very low blood pressure." He shook his head. "I thought as much."

Sammy drew closer to Dr OsGood. "What does that mean?"

"It confirms that she's likely to be bleeding internally. As I discussed with my assistant, she might have a ruptured ectopic pregnancy or any other surgical condition. You may never know till you open her up."

Sammy was confounded. "Does it mean that she had been pregnant?"

"Taking in the scenario of pregnancy, yes. That also means that the baby would appear to be growing in the tubes rather than in the womb." He stopped talking briefly and looked at Sammy. "Other scenarios are also possible."

"Do whatever needs to be done to save her life," Sammy stated.

At that point, Dr OsGood began to issue further instructions.

"Sister Kate, take Mr Sammy to the Medical Records, let them obtain from him as much information as we can get for his wife. Also advise the clerical officers to present an Adult Consent Form to him. We'll discuss it as soon as his wife is ready for surgery."

Sister Kate beckoned Sammy to follow her. Both walked out of the cubicle and through the door opposite cubicle 10 into the hallway which led to the Medical Records department.

Dr OsGood then shifted his attention to Sister Angelina, "Go and arrange the theatre now."

"I'll collect the Consent Form on my way?" Sister Angelina volunteered.

"Yeah, you're right. Drop it off to me in theatre. We'll discuss it along the line. I'll prefer to discuss it with her and her husband."

"Thanks." Sister Angelina announced and left the cubicle.

By this time, Pascal who had gone to park the car, rushed back into the cubicle.

"Hello Mr Pascal, please head to the Medical Records. Mr Sammy is there." Dr OsGood advised.

Pascal left the area as quick as his legs could carry him.

Dr OsGood punched the monitor to verify how her vital signs were going.

He turned to his assistant, "This young lady is not doing well. She has received a bag of normal saline and the second bag is running in. She still has low blood pressure."

"At least the systolic is improving," Dr DoLittle commented.

"You're absolutely right. Note, it's just a marginal improvement. Her heart rate is still high and pulse pressure is narrowing."

Dr DoLittle shuffled his feet. "Do you think that we can commence blood transfusion now?" He asked.

"My guess is yes. We may struggle to stabilise her more than this. We need to identify where she is bleeding from, and it needs to be taken care of as soon as possible."

"That's right," Dr DoLittle affirmed.

"Blood transfusion and her surgery should go hand-in-hand otherwise, she might not make it."

Looking squarely at his superior, Dr DoLittle asked, "What do you want me to do now?"

Dr OsGood approached Abigail, gently touched her on the shoulder. Abigail opened her eyes.

"Are you happy if we wheel you into the theatre? You seem to be bleeding internally."

Abigail nodded.

"I know that you won't have the strength to sign the form. I'll get your husband to sign on your behalf. Are you happy with that?"

Abigail nodded again.

"Please DoLittle, ring her husband and ask him to meet us in the theatre. We'll want him to sign the Consent Form."

Dr OsGood began to step away from the cubicle. "Dr DoLittle, I'm going to the theatre now, so I'll see you in there."

"I'll organise the Consent form, bloods and other essentials before meeting you in the theatre," Dr DoLittle responded.

Dr OsGood left the Emergency room for the theatre at that instant.

As he was walking out, two junior nurses walked in.

"Nurse Mercy, please, I want you to go to Medical Records, pick up Mr Sammy Petters there and advise him that he is needed in the theatre immediately. I'll want you to take him and show him where to wait for Dr OsGood."

"Thanks, I'll do so." Nurse Mercy replied and left the Emergency department.

Dr DoLittle turned to the other nurse, "Annie, we need to prepare Mrs Petters for theatre."

The nurse nodded and waited for further instructions.

"Are you able to insert a catheter?"

"Yes."

"Insert the catheter, give our patient preop medication, and then call a porter who'll transfer her to the theatre as soon as possible."

"Is there anything else that you would want me to do?" Nurse Annie asked.

"Please ring the blood bank and advise them to transfer two to four units of bloods to the theatre immediately."

As Dr DoLittle was walking to the theatre, he met Nurse Mercy and Sammy in the hallway. "Dr OsGood will want to discuss your wife's Consent Form with you. Do you mind following me so that I can take you to him?"

Sammy followed Dr DoLittle and they only walked a short distance from where they met before they ran into Dr OsGood.

"Hello again Mr Petters," Dr OsGood greeted him.

"How are you again, Doc?" Sammy responded.

"I'm fine. If you wouldn't mind, we'll talk as we walk to the changing room. We don't have a lot of time."

Before he could continue his discussion with Sammy, Dr DoLittle handed him some sheets of paper. He stopped briefly and went through the reports.

"As I was saying, your wife is still gravely unwell, and time is ticking away. The report in front of me confirms that she is pregnant. That means that ectopic pregnancy is the likely cause of her bleeding."

At this instant, his phone rang. He stopped, looked at the caller ID and turned to Sammy, "Please permit me to answer it. It's from the Anaesthetist."

Sammy waved in acceptance to him.

"I am, as we speak, walking into the changing room." Dr OsGood replied to the caller. "I need to consent the next of kin before we can get started." He then switched off the phone.

At that point he opened the theatre door and all of them walked in with Dr DoLittle stepping in before them.

As he stepped in, Dr DoLittle informed Dr OsGood, "I'll change into my theatre gowns quickly. And I'll see you in the operating room."

Dr OsGood waved at him and returned his focus to Sammy. He ushered Sammy into the first room, where they both sat down. He then continued his discussion, "Your wife has consented to having an operation. By Law, she is supposed to sign the Consent Form." He placed the form on the table for Sammy to see.

Sammy glanced through the form very hastily or rather absent-mindedly, and then shoved it back across the table to DrOsGood.

"I know you're in significant distress and would want this operation done as soon as possible." He paused and cast a glance at Sammy. "Do you want me to run through the operation procedure and content of the Consent Form for you?"

"You can do so as long as it won't consume a lot of time," Sammy replied reluctantly.

Dr OsGood continued, "We need to open her tummy, identify which tube is housing the embryo. We will then tie it and scoop the baby out. It will be a case that we will need to start her on a blood transfusion at the same time." He ceased to talk as noise was emanating from the floor.

Dr OsGood looked under the table and noticed it was Sammy's toes that created the noise. Apparently, he had been digging the floor all through the discussion with Dr OsGood. "Is everything all right with you?" Dr OsGood asked with great concern.

"Sorry for the noise. I unconsciously dig the floor with my toes when I'm significantly stressed."

"I get it," Dr OsGood commented. "I'll take care of your wife. She'll be fine and I'll talk to you and her after the operation." Dr OsGood then ran off into the Doctors' change room.

With tears pouring down his face, Sammy nodded and waved at Dr OsGood. "I trust you'll save her for me," he screamed out.

Immediately he completed the sentence, the theatre doors whipped open and he peered out of the room where he was sitting and noticed Abigail on a stretcher, being wheeled in.

As the stretcher was reaching the door of the room where he was sitting, Dr DoLittle and the theatre nurses came out from the operating room to receive Abigail. "Do you want to wish your wife good luck?" he asked.

"Sure," Sammy replied still seated. He was confused and wasn't sure how to wish her good luck.

Sister Angelina walked in through the open theatre door at the same time. "Mr Petters, go and give her a gentle kiss," she encouraged.

Sammy, in a dazed state wobbled to the side of the stretcher and placed a firm kiss on Abigail's cheek. "If you die, take me with you," he whispered into her ear.

Sister Angelina heard his comment and felt for him. "She'll not die."

The theatre nurses took over the care of Abigail and they wheeled her into the operating room.

A short while later, Dr OsGood came out clad in a green gown and hat, and from there he entered the operating room.

Chapter 9

Room 25
Life Matters Best Hospital
No 40 Georgina Avenue
Groenkloof 0281, Pretoria
South Africa
April 16, 1986, Wednesday, 9.00 am

Sammy's large hands gently and slowly parted the double-breasted curtain shielding the window on the sixth floor where Abigail's room was located. As he did so, he peered down on people traversing the streets adjacent to the hospital and wondered if any were or had been in the predicament that he was in yesterday. He took a very long and deep breath in a bid to either jettison or block the events from reaching his conscious mind. The more he tried, the more the events loomed larger in his mind; and the more it occurred to him that he didn't know how he had survived it all.

The ordeal started on a very rocky and traumatising note but ended positively, due to the professionalism exhibited by Dr Simon OsGood and his team. He's eternally grateful and indebted to him and his team for the great work they did on Abigail. They saved Abigail's life and invariably his.

The recollection of the theatre ordeal was still haunting him and was very vivid in his mind...

He was left in one of the rooms of the theatre alone after Dr OsGood and his team had gone in to perform Abigail's laparotomy. He sat as if glued to the chair till his bottom became as hard as a rock. He stood up and began to pace around till his feet became very heavy and couldn't move anymore. All along his eyes got fixated on the clock on the opposite wall counting minutes and hours waiting for Abigail to be wheeled out. It looked like it was an eternity.

"Mr Petters wake up," Sister Angelina shook him back to life. "The operation is over, and she is fine," he remembered her telling him.

He didn't know when he'd dozed off or how long he'd been asleep. Apparently, he was found lying on one of the sofa chairs.

When he came around all he wanted was to see Abigail. "She hasn't come out of Recovery yet," the same Sister Angelina informed him.

He got a bit irked and wondered why she woke him up if they were not wheeling Abigail out yet.

As he was beginning to pace around again, his phone rang and when he looked at the caller ID it was Uncle Goddy's number.

"Hello Uncle," he replied.

"How's Abigail's operation?" he asked and went on to inform him that Pascal came back and narrated everything to him. He wanted to wait till the operation was over before he rang him.

"They just informed me that the operation is over and that she's okay, but they've not wheeled her out. So, I've not seen her yet."

"They'll soon do that," he recalled Uncle Goddy reassuring him.

"I don't know if I should believe them or not," he replied to Uncle Goddy.

"You have to believe them."

As Uncle Goddy was trying to convince him that Abigail was okay and that he should exercise some patience, the door to the room where he was opened. "Uncle, I'll call you back soon," he told Uncle Goddy and switched off his phone to attend to the person who was walking in to see him.

"Abigail is out and ready to meet you," Sister Angelina advised him.

He glanced at the clock and the time was 11.00 pm. He flicked his head in utter dismay. The operation had lasted more than three hours. Thank goodness that it's all over now and she is out, he told himself.

He took a deep breath and braced himself to walk out to the stretcher, and was surprised to notice that Abigail had her eyes closed just as she had when she was in distress, before the operation. The difference was that she wasn't however writhing in pain. For a brief moment panic took over. He leapt to the side of her stretcher, "Darling are you all right?"

Abigail slowly opened her eyes and gave him a smile. "I'm a lot better now," she mumbled.

He bent down, began to sob and held Abigail tightly till the nurse tapped him. "Let her go, she just had a major operation."

He let her go and then stood beside the stretcher with his left hand on Abigail's head, stroking her hairs.

"We'll be transferring her to Room 25 where she'll stay till she's discharged from the hospital."

Sister Angelina walked briskly beyond Abigail to the entrance of the theatre and yelled at the orderly,

"Adair, where're you? The patient is ready to be transferred to her room."

"Sorry Sister, I just went to ease myself," he said apologetically.

"Let's go," Sister Angelina commanded.

Adair wheeled the stretcher, with Sister Angelina on one side and Sammy on the other side.

As they were about to walk out of the theatre, Sammy heard somebody walking to them. He turned around and noticed it was Dr OsGood. "How was the op Doc?"

"It was difficult but there was no complication."

"Thanks a lot," he told Dr OsGood.

"That's okay; I'll talk to you people tomorrow when Abigail will have recovered completely from the anaesthesia."

"See you tomorrow then," Sammy responded and continued to their Room 25 with the others.

Apparently, Room 25 was located just a distance further away from the Nurses Station attached to that floor. So, as they were approaching Room 25, Sister Angelina rang other nurses in the Nurses Station and asked them to join her in Abigail's room so that she could do a handover to them there.

Four nurses were already inside Room 25 when Abigail was wheeled in. Immediately they entered, Sister Angina, Orderly Adair and the other nurses joined hands and transferred Abigail onto her bed.

Sister Angelina began to do a handover to the other nurses during which she discussed Abigail's pre and post-operative conditions and while she was doing that, Sammy was busy reviewing the room, his eyes shifting from ceiling to floor and from one end of the wall to the other...

The room was painted blue; was larger and neater than Sammy had imagined. It was roughly 16 mm by 16 mm in dimension; it was pristinely clean and nicely scented with a vase of beautiful rose flowers sitting on a table at the extreme right end corner of the room. A 42 inch TV was tugged at the other end of the room, and adjacent to it was a green curtain covering the window on the east end of the room which prevented light penetrating into the room. Abigail's bed had a brown and white bedspread. It also had a bed scarf. It had adjustable knobs with which the bed's head and foot could be raised or dropped as one wished to do. There was a knob attached to the bedside and an isolated remote control. On the head of her bed were a heart monitor, and an IV drip set. There was another bed which was not so exquisitely decorated as that of Abigail's. This second bed was of king-size and was positioned under the only window in the room. It was obvious that the second bed was for a patient's relative like himself. There were buzzers around the room – one attached to the head of Abigail's bed, the other on the wall and another in the restroom. There was a split air conditioner strategically positioned on the wall directly opposite the door of the restroom. When it was switched on, the air would flow into the restroom.

The restroom, which was attached to Room 25 was reasonably equipped with handrail, moderate sized bathtub, bathroom with a shower, and toilet seat with a standard toilet bowl.

A door was aligned close to the restroom. It led into the kitchenette which had a small refrigerator, a microwave oven with hotplate, and a sink.

There were two buzzers; one on the wall close to the handrail attached to the toilet seat, and the other positioned between the bathtub and shower.

The floor of the restroom was tiled, whereas that in the main room had vinyl. The ceilings of both the main room and restroom were painted yellow. The paint on the ceiling had no visible wear suggesting that it had been recently repainted.

"Mr Petters, we've finished with our handover," Sister Angelina's voice jerks him back into reality.

"Okay, much appreciated."

Sister Angelina stepped forward from where she was and moved closer to Sammy. "Mr Petters, as you'd know, my shift is over so I'm going. Before I go, I need to introduce the nurses who'll be in charge of your wife tonight. They're already aware of her medical condition. They'll do routine checks on her throughout the night." She halted, cleared her throat and continued.

"Although there are four now, only three will be available for the night for you people. Sister Sarah is the leader." She pointed to Sister Sarah at the far-right of Sammy.

"Hello Mr Petters, how are you doing?" Sister Sarah greeted.

"I'm okay Sister Sarah. Please feel free to call me Sammy which is my first name."

"Note taken," Sister Sarah responded.

"The second in command, if I may use such a word is Sister Vickie," Sister Angelina pointed to her.

"Hello Sammy, are you okay?" Sister Vickie said.

"I'm fine. Hope you're fine also."

Sister Angelina shifted a bit to face the third nurse. "This is Sister Emma."

Sister Emma exchanged pleasantries with Sammy as the others had done.

"Before I step away, it may also be necessary to inform you that the night nurses will check Abigail every hour for the next four hours, then they'll do that two-hourly till morning, then ..."

As she was commenting, Abigail began to moan. "Are you in pain?" Sister Angelina asked her.

"Yeah," Abigail replied softly.

"We'll get you pain relief very soon," Sister Sarah replied and beckoned the others to follow her, and they all began to walk out of the room.

"Good night, Sammy and Mrs Petters," Sister Angelina commented. "I'll see you tomorrow."

"Thanks for all your help," Sammy responded. "Have a good sleep for the rest of the night."

It wasn't long before Sister Sarah and Sister Vickie came back, each clutching a kidney dish in their hands.

"I want to give you a morphine injection under the skin of your tummy," Sister Sarah stated. "Are you happy if I do so?" She asked Abigail.

"Yeah, go ahead."

"Protocol requires us to ask you for a confirmation of your identity too."

Abigail slowly opened her eyes and stated, "I'm Mrs Abigail Petters. My date of birth is June 5th, 1960."

Sister Sarah turned to her colleague, "Are you satisfied with her confirmation?"

"Yeah, I am."

Sister Sarah swabbed Abigail's abdomen and gave her the injection. "Immediately you begin to feel pain, press your PCA." She pointed out to Abigail the tiny needle inserted on the other side of her tummy. "Of course, press the buzzer if it's too excruciating."

"I'm grateful," Abigail murmured.

Shifting her focus to Sammy who had already made himself comfortable on the bed, "Please, you can press the buzzer for her at any time, if either of you are concerned. We'll come rushing in."

"You people have been marvellous," Sammy responded.

The two nurses bade Sammy and Abigail goodnight and left their room to go back to their Nurses Station...

A tap on their door woke Sammy up. "How's your wife?" Sister Sarah asks?

"She has not moaned in pain since the last injection she received around 5.00 am." He looked at Abigail who had begun to writhe in bed. "I think she is in pain now, so she might need some injection again."

"Okay, I'll grab another injection for her now." As she was leaving the room, she turned around and said, "I should be able to give her the injection before I start handover, otherwise it'll be time for the morning shift nurses and they will be able to do it. My shift will end at 7.30 am."

"Thanks for being considerate and helpful." Sammy commended her.

Sammy looked at his watch, it's already 7.00 am. "I've not slept a wink." And then he threw himself back to his bed.

It was not long before the nurse came back with Sister Vickie, both walking serenely and purposefully. They went through the same ritual before they administered the injection.

As Sammy was about to doze off, his phone rang. He looked at the caller ID. "Hello Uncle Goddy, how are you?" he muttered.

"I'm fine," Uncle Goddy responded. "How's Abigail?"

"They just gave her an injection. She slept well last night."

"How does she look?"

"At least she is able to talk now, although softly. She is brighter."

"How was last night?"

"I would've said it was hitch-free, but it wasn't."

Uncle Goddy hissed and sounded alarmed over the phone. "What happened?"

"It was around 4.00 am when she moaned, became restless and tried to climb out of her bed."

"What was the cause of her restlessness?" Uncle Goddy questioned.

"I quickly pressed the buzzer and they rushed in. After they reviewed her, they told me they suspected that her bladder was full, and she needed to urinate. They called the doctor, who took a bit of time to come …"

Uncle Goddy interrupted him, "So when he came, what did he find?"

"He confirmed what the nurses had already noted. And he re-inserted the catheter. And then the nurses came back and gave her an injection."

"So, both of you slept thereafter?"

"Yeah, she did but I didn't."

"Just digressing to another important topic, you know your dad's burial is today."

Sammy's head dropped, his brain went blank and fogged; and he suddenly felt a pain like a sharp knife was piercing through his heart. He had virtually forgotten about the burial today because of his wife's illness and operation.

He was not responding very fast.

"Are you still there?" Uncle Goddy asked. He too had gotten the clue that Sammy had become distressed again. "I've told the elders that Abigail isn't well and has just had an operation and that you're with her in the hospital."

Trying to recover his composure, "What was their response?" Sammy queried.

"They all understood." He waited for a response— when none was forthcoming from Sammy he went on. "They've excused you from attending."

"Are all the burial arrangements completed?"

"I would say yes."

As he was saying that Abigail turned her head to make eye contact with Sammy. "Good morning, Uncle Goddy."

"Darling, he can't hear you." Sammy then quickly switched on to speaker. "Repeat yourself now."

"Hello, Uncle Goddy."

"How are you Abigail?"

"I'm getting better," she replied with a voice barely audible.

"That's good. Thank Heavens for your operation. We're sure you'll make a good recovery."

"Thanks Sir. Is the burial still being held today?"

"Yes Abigail. Arrangements have already been finalised for it. The ambulance car that will take his corpse to Brakpan has already been arranged and other burial formalities are already in place."

Abigail was sad, "So it can't be postponed till next week to enable us to partake in it?" She responded in a forlorn voice.

"You know it's the culture. Bodies aren't allowed to be kept for longer than the stipulated cultural time otherwise things could go awry."

Abigail sighed. Sammy did the same. They both looked at each other but uttered no word.

Ghostly silence descended among them. Uncle Goddy too went mum.

"Okay, I've got to go now. I've a few things to sort out. We'll visit you around 5.00 pm today, after the burial," Uncle Goddy stated with a note of finality.

"Bye," they both said.

Abigail closed her eyes again and probably dozed off to sleep and Sammy edged to the head of his bed and through the window continued to watch people walking along the street.

Chapter 10

Life Matters Best Hospital
No 40 Georgina Avenue
Groenkloof 0281, Pretoria
South Africa
April 17, 1986, Thursday, 4.00 pm

Sammy took the lift hoping to reach the hospital kiosk at the ground floor on time so as to buy some cards for Abigail and personal effects for their use. By the time he made it to the door of the kiosk, it had already closed for the day. He didn't know that it shuts at 3.30 pm. As he was contemplating either to ring a taxi and get into town, or return to the room to be with Abigail, he heard a loud noise coming from outside the end of the hospital where cars were parked. It sounded like the roar of a lion or probably like a train, ferrying things along, but when he listened attentively it seemed to be coming from the sky.

He stepped out into the open to decipher the source and cause of the noise; he looked up and had to fix his gaze for some minutes to make out the colours of the sky; closer to the hospital building had a bluish tint and a bit further away had a golden appearance, and in the middle was a greenish-yellow colour. He exhaled long and hard in disbelieve as to what he was seeing; could this be a tornado unfolding? He really does not know much about such natural phenomena.

"Hello, young fellow," a deep baritone voice was heard from behind him. "How are you?"

The voice jolted him. He turned around and responded, "I'm great, and you?"

"I'm fantastic. I've come to visit my niece who had an appendix removed two days ago."

"My wife had an abdominal surgery a day ago," Sammy replied.

"By the way, I'm Rodriguez Junior, having been named after my father. Friends call me Rod for short," he stated with a smile which exposed a set of disjointed grey-looking false dentures.

"I'm Sammy Petters." He then shook hands with Rod who had extended his hand.

Rod appeared as a middle-aged white Caucasian. His age could be somewhere between 65 to 70 years. He had mottled bald with grey-white long hair around its edges which spread onto the sides of his face. When the wind blew, the hairs fluttered into his mouth. He had a pair of round glasses which were hanging on the tip of his nose. Behind the glasses were deep set brown eyes with yellow edges around them signifying advanced cataracts. His face was wrinkled and had a wizened appearance to it. He was wearing whitish-coloured long moustaches which could do with some trimming judging by their length and texture. He was unable to stand straight as his back was slightly hunched.

"It seems you're intrigued by the unfolding weather?" Rod hinted.

"Yes, I am." Sammy looked at him. "What about you? Are you not?"

"I am, from a different perspective though," he paused.

"How do you mean?"

"I've been a tornado chaser all through my life. I was an active chaser in my hay days when I was a lot younger, but do so sparingly these days because of my frailty and age."

Sammy was getting interested in this haggard looking man. He certainly appeared as interesting as the tornados themselves, Sammy told himself.

As they were talking, lightning struck, and the bright light accentuated the wrinkles in the skin of his arms, and also the severity of his unkemptness.

A loud noise was heard again. Then hail in the size of ice cubes, and later like golf balls began to fall from the sky. Initially they fell singularly and then within the space of seconds in bundles. It was intermixed with thunderstorms. As the hail fell onto car roofs; the latter became drums for the music which ensued. The fall of the hails onto the cars could be likened to a musical rhythm with the car roofs as the drum for the drummer.

Rod tapped Sammy, "Let's get inside. I think the worst of this weather is yet to come. Otherwise we might get caught up with the havoc which runs in its trail if it develops into a tornado," he paused. "That's if it eventuates into one."

Both men began walking back into the hall way.

"Do you really think that this will eventuate into a tornado?" Sammy asked.

"Emphatically," Rod started, "Even the most intelligent of the meteorologists mightn't be able to answer this question with certainty."

"Why is it so?"

"Because it's an act of nature." Rod grinned. "Nature most often doesn't disclose all that is in its baggage."

Sammy was keen on continuing the discussion on tornadoes. "So, tell me more, what signs could predict the arrival of tornadoes?"

Rod cleared his throat, "I could give you about six or seven atmospheric warning signs that precipitate a tornado's arrival."

"Could dark or greenish or golden colour of the sky be some of those?" Sammy asked.

"Yeah, you're on the ball. Others would be wall clouds or what appears like an approaching cloud of debris."

Sammy nodded and in a bid to contribute to the discussion made further suggestions. "Would large hail which might occur in the absence of rain be another important one?"

"Again yes, it seems that you've a fair idea of tornadoes and their precipitating signs."

They were already on the sixth floor. They both stepped out of the lift and Sammy decided to pursue the discussion.

"I just want to make a reasonable assessment if there might be tornadoes tonight."

"If you must; the other signs could be that before a tornado strikes, the wind might have died down and the air might've become still." Rod was happy to deliver more lectures.

"Despite all that I've analysed for you this evening and the great strides already made in meteorology that help and guide us to understand and predict tornadoes, there are still many unknown variables. So, the only certainties are advance warning and proper precaution."

"Are there specific times that tornadoes would likely strike?"

"Again, without meaning to act as God, tornadoes can arrive at any hour, but they usually strike during late afternoon and early evening, such as from 3.00 pm to 9.00 pm."

"How many tornadoes were you able to catch during your time?"

"About five only; because they display the beastly side of Mother Nature and if you're caught up in it you're a goner." He paused to answer his phone which had beeped.

Sammy gazed at him.

"It's a text message from one of my granddaughters asking where I was."

"In which room is your niece and grand-children?"

Pointing to the other side of the hallway, just two rooms down that side, "I think that's room 23," he stated.

Sammy raised his right thumb and pointed behind them, "That's where we are, that's room 25."

"The two rooms are certainly close to each other."

"Can we go in so that you can say hello to my wife?"

"Sure, let's do so."

As they turned around Sammy noticed that Abigail had stood up from where she was sitting and was about to walk out to join them on the veranda.

Sammy went to the Nurses Station and asked for three chairs for the three of them.

Sammy was glad that she was not lying down anymore and was able to come out. "Darling, how are you?" he asked.

"A lot better today. I've not needed any morphine injections since this afternoon."

"It means that your pain is resolving."

"Yeah," Abigail affirmed.

"Darling, this is Mr Rod, for short. He used to be a tornado chaser."

Sammy turned to Rod. "My wife's name is Abigail."

Both Rod and Abigail exchanged pleasantry. They also shook hands with each other.

"Rod has been teaching me about the tornadoes, since we met a short while ago."

"Hello Rod, are tornadoes common natural disasters?"

"They're certainly not although there are records of them in history."

Sammy was elated at seeing his wife appearing well again. He drew closer and put his hand around her shoulders. "He told me that he has been able to catch five tornadoes during his time. He also knows a lot of the warning signs in the weather which will depict the arrival of a tornado."

"Have you had tornadoes here in South Africa?" Abigail queried.

"There have been about five since 1948."

Abigail and Sammy were enrapt with the discussion.

"Can you give us a breakdown of the events?" Sammy requested.

"The first was named Roodepoort. The records have it that it happened in Highveld on 26 November 1948. There were 14 recorded fatalities, about 101 injuries and about 705 homes destroyed."

"That's an interesting piece of history." Abigail was certainly amazed. "When was the last one?"

"The last one was named Trompsburg tornado and noted to have occurred in Karoo around 5 November 1976. It consumed five lives and its longest measured path was 175 km."

"Are there countries worst hit by tornadoes more often?" Sammy asked.

"I'm unable to give an answer to that because I'm not a good historian but I know they've hit eight times in my country of birth."

Abigail became inquisitive, "Which country are you talking about here?"

"Argentina. The first one occurred in 1816, consuming 21 lives and 82 injuries in its trail. The worst of all occurred in 1973 in Santa Fe Province. It resulted in 63 fatalities."

As they were still conversing, Abigail noted, "It's news time. They'll likely give us a weather forecast update soon."

A short while later, as Abigail came back with the radio, an announcement was being made:

"The revised forecast for today's weather is along these lines: heavy rain showers for Pretoria and Gauteng areas; and there will also be a two-faced storm to end as heavy snowfall across most other parts of the Northeast. The visibility is predicated to be around 8 km. The predicted daytime temperature is going to reach 33 °c and will dip to 17 °c at night. Annabel for the Bureau of Mets- SA."

Shortly after they heard the weather forecast, Sammy's phone rang. He picked it up and looked at the caller ID. "It's Uncle Goddy," he announced. "Hold on Uncle."

At the same time, Rod's own phone rang and he picked up. "I'm on my way," he told the caller. He then stood up. "They need me now," he stated and waved at Abigail and Sammy and left.

Sammy stood up and beckoned to Abigail for them to go inside. He switched his phone to speaker.

Sammy was very apologetic. "Sorry Uncle for keeping you waiting. It wasn't intentional. We had a visitor but he's gone now."

"Not a problem," Uncle Goddy replied. "How are you people?"

"We're fine. Abigail is recovering very well." Sammy replied.

"We've just finished with the burial now."

"How did it go?" Abigail asked.

"It was a success," he replied. "Geraldine and my wife are in the car with me. They can hear you."

"Mum, how are you?" Sammy asked.

"I would say okay." She replied and began to sob.

"Stop crying. He's gone. You tried your best." Abigail advised.

"We'll try and console her," Uncle Goddy's wife reassured them.

"We've just left Brakpan some 10 minutes ago. It'll take us another 50 minutes to get into Pretoria. We'll come to the hospital to see you people immediately we are back," Uncle Goddy informed them.

Sammy wanted to make sure that they avoid certain highways, "Which route are you travelling through?"

"We'll be going via Ben Schoeman Freeway and Pretoria Main Rd/N1."

"That seems safe," Sammy reassured them.

"We'll hope to be with you people by 5.30 pm."

"We'll see you when you get here," both Abigail and Sammy echoed.

They heard a knock on their door. "Come on in," Abigail called.

Sister Angelina walked in with some morphine in a kidney dish. She was followed by her assistant Sister Vickie who had a thermometer and stethoscope.

"Hello Mrs Petters, we're here to administer your 4.30 pm morphine injection," Sister Angelina announced.

Abigail smiled and sat upright in her chair. "Sorry Sisters, I don't want any more injections."

"Why don't you want it?" Sister Vickie asked.

"My pain is reasonably controlled as of now, and moreover the morphine makes me feel funny."

Sister Angelina lent her voice to the discussion, "That's okay. Some say it makes them throw up and others, it makes them hallucinate."

"It also gives me hallucinations."

"Then it's reasonable to remove it from your list of medications." Sister Angelina concluded. "Hope you'll be happy to be prescribed oral pain tablets?"

"Of course, I'm okay with oral medications." Abigail confirmed.

"Sister Vickie, could you administer the oral tablet in your possession?"

"Sure," Sister Vickie responded, and handed the medications to Abigail.

Sammy stood up and moved towards the door, "I wonder if it's still raining?"

Sister Vickie had begun to check Abigail's blood pressure and temperature. "It has since dried up," she commented in between the examination.

Immediately Sister Vickie finished examining Abigail, Sammy asked, "How is she doing?"

"She's doing well. Her BP, temperature and other vitals are within normal range," Sister Vickie remarked as she joined Sister Angelina and they began walking towards the door.

Before they stepped out of Abigail's room, Sister Angelina turned around, "Mrs Petters, Dr OsGood rang and informed us to advise you that he'll be coming to review you by 5.30 pm or sooner than that if he finishes the operation that he is doing."

Abigail's face brightened up. "That's good. Has he been in theatre all throughout today?"

"I would say most of the afternoon, precisely, since 12 midday." Sister Angelina replied.

She and Sister Vickie left Abigail's room.

It wasn't too long after the exit of the nurses that Sammy's phone buzzed. He grabbed it from the desk where it was lying and looked at the caller ID. "Uncle Goddy is here," he commented. And he then put the phone on speaker.

"Hello Uncle, where are you?"

"We're at the ground floor. What's Abigail's room number?"

"She is in room 25." Sammy replied.

"We're getting into the lift now and will be up there soon."

"See you people soon," Sammy and Abigail echoed.

As soon as Sammy dropped the call from Uncle Goddy, there had a knock on their door.

Dr OsGood, Dr DoLittle, Sister Angelina and Sister Vickie walked in.

Dr OsGood reviewed Abigail, "How are you going Mrs Petters?"

"I think that I'm going well."

"Do you mind lying on the bed so that I can examine your abdomen?"

Abigail did as she was asked.

While examining her abdomen, Dr OsGood commented, "It seems that your pain is tolerable." Then he looked up at her. "Or could be you've got a very high pain threshold."

Sammy was watching the scene closely. "It takes a lot for her to complain of pain."

Dr OsGood nodded. "So, your pain is being controlled on oral pain medications only."

"Yeah, besides morphine makes me feel extremely unwell."

"No, we don't want you feeling unwell again," Dr OsGood commented as he was finishing his examination.

Abigail sat up. "What did you find during the operation?" she asked.

"You had an ectopic pregnancy; that is where the baby is developing in one of the tubes rather than in the womb. It often leads to the rupture of the relevant tube. In your case it was your right tube." He stopped and scanned Abigail's face. He wanted to ensure that she comprehended.

"What does it mean for me, going forward?"

"You can get pregnant, but it has to be only through the left tube."

Sammy shifted on his chair and asked. "Is it likely that she would have another ectopic which would affect her left tube in the future?"

"The possibility is there. Having said that, women who have had an ectopic pregnancy often go ahead to achieve normal pregnancy." He paused to see if they had more questions for him.

"When do you think I'll be discharged?" Abigail asked.

"It could be tomorrow or the next day, depending on you."

Sammy stepped in again. "We'll want to go home tomorrow."

"That's fine by me," Dr OsGood responded.

Sammy immediately wore a concerned look. "Can we see you tomorrow?"

"Sure. Is there any problem?" Dr OsGood was worried.

"We'd like to discuss our health problem further and see how it could affect my wife, and how we could have a healthy baby."

"I'll hold the discussion with you people but be informed that I might be retiring very soon. I'm sure Dr DoLittle, my able assistant will still be available to help you people, if I'm gone by the time you want it."

Sammy was elated. "That's okay."

"I'll ask the nurses to inform you tomorrow when I'll come around for the discussion." Dr OsGood commented with a tone of finality.

They all lined up and began to march out as they came in.

Dr OsGood was the last in line to head to the door. As he reached the door, he turned around. "Mr and Mrs Petters, it seems you've visitors who have been waiting for you people."

He walked out and disappeared into the hallway.

Uncle Goddy, his wife and Geraldine walked in. Sammy narrated all that had happened to Abigail, and they in turn updated Abigail and Sammy on how the burial went.

"It's getting very late. We'd rather keep going," Uncle Goddy voiced. "We'll see you tomorrow."

Sammy and Abigail waved at them, "When do we expect you tomorrow?" Abigail asked.

"Around 10 or 11 am." Uncle Goddy replied and waved back.

Chapter 11

Room 25
Life Matters Best Hospital
No 40 Georgina Avenue
Groenkloof 0281, Pretoria
South Africa
April 18, 1986, Friday Morning

Sammy was lying on the hospital bed in Room 25 but was tossing and turning.

∞ ∞

"How're you Sammy?" Mighty M asked.

Sammy was not sure how to reply to his father, "I'm fine," he said reluctantly.

Sammy's body language gave him away. "What's the problem with you?" his father asked.

"I've got terrible right hip pain again which is shooting down into my leg."

Mighty M observed Sammy on the bed for a while and noted that he was struggling to find a comfortable position. "You normally suffer from the right hip pain. Is it worse now?"

"It seems so," Sammy replied. "So why are you here?"

"I just came to see Abigail.". Mighty M then sat down on the sofa chair in the centre of the room. He then crossed his legs.

"Why have you come to see Abigail?" Sammy queried.

"I know she has been in pain. I've come to fix her."

Sammy was confused. 'What do you mean that you've come to fix her?"

Sammy observed his father pull out a bag containing injections. "I've some injections to give her," he affirmed.

"Dad, when did you become a doctor?"

As his father was about to respond, he collapsed and began to have seizures then went limp.

Sammy quickly ducked down and began doing CPR on his father but couldn't resuscitate him and then he began to cry loudly ...

∞ ∞

"Darling what's happening?" Abigail screamed.

Sammy's loud cry had woken her up. Her husband had been resilient, tough and strong but his father's death and her sudden illness had rendered him decrepit.

Sammy leapt up from his bed in alarm when he heard Abigail's scream. "Sorry, I was dreaming," he explained in a feeble voice.

Sammy's sleep last night was thwarted not by the restlessness of his wife, but by his own back and hip pain. The mattress on the bed was very firm and that affected his sleep significantly. In between the bouts of pain, he tried to sleep, and when he did go into a deep sleep, he dreamt of the interaction which he had with his late father.

Abigail felt sad and miserable because of her husband's current state of mind. "What caused you to cry out?"

"It was a horrible dream?"

"What do you mean?"

"I couldn't help him at all?"

"Who couldn't you help?"

"My dad..."

"Darling, please stop speaking in riddles and tell me what you dreamt of." Abigail was exasperated.

Sammy lowered his face and covered it with his hands. "Ahem," he cleared his throat and then went on to narrate his dream to his wife.

Abigail paid rapt attention. When Sammy finished, she commented, "So he had come to save me before his epilepsy hit him?"

"Seems so," Sammy acquiesced. "That's why I felt so bad that I couldn't revive him."

Abigail shrugged her shoulders, "He might've been in the theatre with me when Dr OsGood was operating on me?"

In Abigail's and Sammy's culture, there's a belief in the power of the dead. It's believed that a dead person who liked you might pay you a visit to save you when you're in trouble. Vice-versa they could hunt you and make life miserable for you if you did evil things to them. The spirit world is much revered in their culture.

"I still believe that he'd come to tell us something." Sammy suggested.

Abigail shrugged her shoulders again but this time in a non-committal way, "Probably he came to wish us well and to show us that epilepsy isn't good."

As they were still trying to unravel Sammy's dream, they heard a knock.

Sammy responded, "Come in."

Sister Angelina walked into their room, alone this time.

"How are you Abigail? You're certainly looking a lot better." Sister Angelina observed.

"You're correct."

"I came to enquire if you'll need any injectable pain killer today?"

Abigail has continued to require the Ketorolac injections once or twice per day only, no longer on regular basis. She'd, however, stopped receiving Morphine injections.

"No, I won't need them anymore thanks," Abigail replied.

Sister Angelina settled down and carried out her observations. She then looked up, "Your vital signs are normal."

"That's great news." Abigail responded.

As Sister Angelina was about to leave their room, "Since you're not requiring injections anymore, in that case, do you want me to cancel you from our patients' lists that do require injectable analgesics?

"I guess so."

"I've also come to tell you that Dr OsGood rang and advised that he'll come around to review you around 11.00 am today."

Sammy sprang up. "Does it mean that she may be discharged today?" he asked.

"Certainly, your wife is looking good. She has responded very well to her treatment and has made a good recovery. So, I see no reason for keeping her longer than she is supposed to stay."

"Does it mean that I'll go today?" Abigail pressed on.

"The decision is for Dr OsGood to make but I believe he'll let you home today," having said that, she headed for the door.

"Bye nurse," Abigail said and bade her farewell. Sammy did also.

Immediately that Sister Angelina shut the door behind her, Sammy wriggled into Abigail's bed and cuddled her.

"Darling, do you make anything out of my dream?"

Abigail straightened her neck, "Your dad had a message for us."

Sammy squinted his eyes and zeroed into thinking mood. "Would his message relate to his death or to us?"

"I'd believe that his appearance in your dream relates to us more than to his death," Abigail responded.

Sammy's thoughts had always been on his family history of epilepsy. He'd of late, come to the conclusion that they'll need some form of genetic selection, or avoidance, in order for their children to avert having it.

Sammy nodded. "That's my thought process also."

"What then are you thinking?" Abigail quizzed him.

Sammy sat up. "If I were to interpret his message for us, it would be that we need to discuss epilepsy and ways to prevent our babies from contracting it."

Silence fell between them. It seemed Sammy was cogitating about what he'd just said and Abigail on her own part seemed to be contemplating the relevance of Sammy's interpretation.

Sammy untangled himself from Abigail, "Probably, we should broach this topic with Dr OsGood when he comes in today," he commented as he stepped into the kitchenette to make some coffee.

Abigail agreed. "You're right. We should do that."

"Do you want a cup of coffee?"

"Sure, I do. Thanks," Abigail indicated as she was reviewing her abdominal wound.

Sammy glanced at the clock. "It's already 10.30 am."

"So, we'll be expecting Dr OsGood soon." Abigail observed as she was enjoying the hot cup of coffee which her husband had delivered to her. "You should've been a barista!"

Sammy smiled. "Probably, I'll attend a catering school when we get back home."

As they were still talking, Sammy peeped through the window. "I think I see Uncle Goddy and mum stepping out of the car."

"So, your sight is so good that you could make out Uncle Goddy from a distance." Abigail commented.

"Yeah, my sight is always good..."

"But your hips ain't," his wife completed the sentence for him.

"Probably my right hip and leg are bad."

It wasn't long before they heard a knock on the door.

"Come on in," Sammy announced and rushed to open the door.

Uncle Goddy; Chelsea, his wife; Geraldine, Sammy's mother and Pascal, their driver walked in.

"How're you today?" Uncle Goddy asked focusing his gaze at Abigail.

Abigail smiled, "I'm ready to go home."

"Meaning that you've fully recovered?" Geraldine asked.

"I won't say fully recovered." She paused but continued, "Reasonably recovered to be allowed home." Abigail concluded.

"Seems you're bored here," Pascal chucked in.

Abigail took a deep breath. "You can say that again."

Sammy watched his mother intently, "How was last night?"

Geraldine sighed. "It was okay."

"Do you want to know the truth; she didn't sleep a wink," asserted Chelsea.

"She cried her eyes out and probably her heart too," chipped in Uncle Goddy.

On hearing that, Sammy's face dropped, and Abigail suddenly felt unwell.

Uncle Goddy appreciated the body languages of Sammy and his wife. "Has Dr OsGood been here today to see you?" he asked in order to diffuse the tension and change the topic.

"No, he hasn't," replied Abigail.

"We're expecting him soon," Sammy said.

As they were conversing Sammy's phone rang. He picked up and as usual glanced at the caller's ID.

"Who is it?" Abigail asked him.

"It's Sergeant Bet," he replied.

"Put the phone on speaker."

Sammy did as he was told. "Hello Sergeant Bet. How are you?"

"I'm great. How's your wife?"

"She's doing well." Sammy looked at Abigail motioning her to make a comment. "She's listening."

"Oh, right." Sergeant Bet sounded a bit alarmed. "Mrs Petters, how's your health now?"

"I'm fantastic."

"Sorry, I've not been able to come in to see you. The tornado that came in yesterday prevented me making it to the hospital. I was on the way to you when it started, so I went back."

Abigail was quite impressed that Sergeant Bet had made an effort to see her yesterday. "I'm grateful for the attempt."

"Any news for us?" Sammy asked.

"Certainly, the driver confessed and in so doing gave us vital information into the operation of the criminal ring." She paused to answer another phone. "I shall be back in few minutes."

Sammy and Abigail waited patiently till she came back online.

"As I was saying, he was given mitigated gaol term for confessing. The judge also ruled that some money be released to you from the Victims Impact purse."

Sammy had become fidgety and was digging the floor with his feet. "You wouldn't know how much we could be expecting?"

"No, sorry, I don't know. That would have to be worked out by the Department of Justice."

"We're just trying to figure out how we'll go back to our Bloemfontein home when my wife is discharged."

"The good news for you and your wife is that because there's an approved fund waiting to be disbursed, the Insurance Company will be eager to give you a loan car to use till the fund is ready."

"So, what next from here?" asked Abigail.

"The Department will ring you or your husband when the fund is ready for collection."

Sammy was relieved. "Thanks for the information. It is good."

"Thanks Mr and Mrs Petters. May I head off now? I've another duty to attend to."

"Sure. Thanks once more for the help you rendered." Sammy and Abigail echoed. Sergeant Bet dropped off thereafter.

Abigail's alarm went off. She had the alarm to remind her when to take her medications.

"It's already 11.30 am," she muttered as she picked up her watch. She then proceeded getting her medications from the bedside drawer.

They then heard a knock on their door.

"Come in," Sammy sang out.

The door swung open. Dr OsGood, Dr DoLittle, and Sister Angelina marched in.

The trio exchanged greetings with the Petters family.

Dr OsGood sat opposite Abigail, "How are you doing today?"

Abigail beamed with smiles. "I think I'm ready to be discharged."

"That's great news," responded Dr OsGood. "May I request that you people leave the room so that I can examine Mrs Petters."

Everyone except Sammy and the medical team stood up and left the room.

Dr OsGood then proceeded to examine Abigail and at the end confirmed that her abdominal wound was healing very well. "Yes, I'll be happy to discharge you," he confirmed.

Sister Angelina drew closer to Abigail. "We'll organise your take home medications before you leave."

"You shouldn't get pregnant for the next six months, because one of the medications which you'll be given is destructive to unborn babies." Dr OsGood cautioned.

Abigail was uncomfortable. "Is it the medication given to prevent me from having another ectopic?"

"You're correct." Dr OsGood responded. He then turned around to his assistant, "Dr DoLittle can you please organise her scripts and review date."

"Where will we review her? Will it be in Pretoria or in Bloemfontein?" Dr DoLittle asked his Boss.

Dr OsGood shifted his focus to Abigail, "We also run outreach clinics in Bloemfontein. Will you want us to see you there?"

"Sure, it'll be much easier for me."

"That's settled then. We'll see you there in three weeks," Dr OsGood confirmed.

As Dr OsGood was about to leave the room, Sammy tapped him on the shoulder, "Doc, we've some medical problems we want to discuss with you."

Dr OsGood sat back down and advised Dr DoLittle also to stay put. "You can go back to your Nurses Station," he advised Sister Angelina.

After the doctors sat back, Sammy narrated how his father battled with epilepsy all his life and eventually succumbed to it when he was drowned in the bathtub when he had a seizure.

"We'll want to have a baby whose genes will be screened so that he or she won't develop epilepsy." He paused and waited for a response from Dr OsGood.

Dr OsGood immediately wriggled his body and sat upright. "Do you mean gene manipulation to get rid of an epilepsy carrying gene?"

"Yeah, you're right. Can it be done?"

Dr OsGood shifted his focus between Sammy and Abigail, "Modern medicine is capable of a lot of things."

Abigail sat up from her bed and asked, "How successful would such a procedure be?"

"Mrs Petters, it's difficult to give a precise answer to your question because there are variety genetic abnormalities that cause epilepsy. Do you want me to take you through most of them?"

"Certainly, as long as you don't make it very technical," Sammy confirmed.

"From animal studies carried out, the most common epilepsy genes were ion-channel related. This accounted for 28 of the 84 epilepsy genes. It meant that mutations in ion-channel genes would produce a variety of epilepsies with differing phenotypes ranging from mild to severe."

Sammy was nodding as Dr OsGood was explaining. Abigail being a teacher appreciated that abnormalities of ion-channel had something to do with epilepsy.

"What gene, or gene mutations are involved in ion-channel regulation?" asked Abigail.

"It's the mutations in the GABRA1 gene. Its runs show strongly when present in form referred to as autosomal dominant pattern."

"What does that mean?" Sammy asked.

"It means that one copy of the altered gene in each cell is sufficient to cause the disorder."

Abigail had done some research. "What about the inheritance pattern for the so-called juvenile myoclonic epilepsy; what gene mutation causes it?"

"It is believed to be related to mutations in the EFHC1 gene, although this is not certain."

"How will this gene manipulation be achieved?" Sammy quizzes him.

"It'll be done through IVF."

Abigail desired to leap into the unknown, "If it fails what'll be the next available option?"

"You could manage the epilepsy with medications and if that fails then there's an option for brain surgery."

"How successful is brain surgery?" Abigail questioned.

"It is reasonably successful," Dr OsGood stated.

Dr DoLittle decided to contribute. "There are still some chances of failure during the brain surgery."

"We know." Sammy confirmed. "It depends on how it's done and how lucky the patient is."

"You got it right exactly," Dr DoLittle affirmed.

Dr OsGood believes that he has given Mr and Mrs Petters enough information to guide them. "Let us know if you want to go ahead with the IVF procedure after six months."

"We'll go ahead with it," both Sammy and Abigail confirmed.

"Okay, we'll see you then." Dr OsGood stood and beckoned his assistant to do so. "I'll see you during the review, and Dr DoLittle will ring you a week before to remind you."

Sammy was grateful. "Thanks for all your help and for explaining this IVF process to us."

Dr OsGood and Dr DoLittle left Abigail's room.

After they left, Uncle Goddy and the others came back in.

Michael and his wife Agnes had arrived by this time. They came in with Uncle Goddy.

"Sammy and Abigail, you two will ride back with Michael and Agnes, whereas the rest of us will be driven back by Pascal." He paused to make sure that they understood him. "Abigail please, pack your things and collect your scripts and drugs. I'll go and pay the hospital bill."

Sammy turned to Abigail and stated, "Now, understand that Uncle Goddy organised all the executive treatment that we got, and he has also decided to pay the bills."

They both thanked Uncle Goddy profusely and proceeded to get ready to leave the hospital, while Uncle Goddy went downstairs to sort out the bills.

Chapter 12

The Little Paradise Child Care
No 10 O'Leary Avenue
Bloemfontein, Orange Free State
South Africa
September 22, 1990, Saturday Morning

The situation has become much more tensed in Bloemfontein and in most parts of Pretoria since Thursday morning, two days ago, after the protests broke out.

In the middle of O'Leary Street, Sammy's car was sandwiched in between two groups of rioters. Behind them the protesting was still active: they could hear rioters howling in anger; some jeering and others shouting at the tops of their voices. They heard windows being smashed.

In front of them, the rioting did not seem to be as active. In a split second the crowd that had been screaming and cheering went silent, and as they watched the rioters, some wearing masks took to their heels. They dashed off the main street into smashed buildings. They dissipated as fast as they had appeared.

Sammy and Abigail sat in their car watching the events in utter disbelief.

"These rioters have become irate mindless and dangerous mobs who'll knock the sense out of anyone who dares try to stop them," Sammy commented.

As they were watching Police approached them, "Move your car immediately," their leader screamed.

Sammy ignited the car and screeched off, dodging the burnt tyres and logs of woods on the road.

He could hear the Police delivering instructions through loud-speakers and then through the rear mirror he saw them unleashed tear gas onto the mobs behind them.

"We're lucky that they didn't set us ablaze," stated Abigail. "It reminds me about the car hijack," she lamented.

"We're indeed fortunate," Sammy confirmed. He went on, "It's tipped to get worse in few days."

As they were driving past the last street, which was barricaded, they saw more Hercules Police anti-riot squads driving into the scene.

"Apparently the Police have called for back-up because they hadn't made any impact, and certainly hadn't brought the situation under control," Sammy noted.

Abigail had broken out in goose bumps, and had become really shaken up. "What are they rioting for?"

"While we were still in the midst of them, I heard their spokes-person allude to the fact that their protest was related to embezzle-ment of tax-payers' money by politicians. And there was poor service deliverance. Roads weren't maintained and when they were, they were done poorly."

"They also were spreading pamphlets which had in bold, that there are no drugs in hospitals; schools are not equipped, and workers are owed arrears in monthly salaries," Abigail chipped in.

It wasn't long before they were completely out of being harmed by the rioters. Abigail looked back and noticing fumes of smoke still going up in the air; she and Sammy heaved a sigh of relief.

Sammy and Abigail had been warned by their neighbour a day ago that they were going to protest in the middle part of their city, and that if they chose to go to their child's Child Care that chances were they might run into the protesters but they decided to risk it as they were intent on giving Guy a befitting first birthday ceremony and weren't eager to postpone it.

Abigail glanced at little Guy in his capsule; he was asleep and appeared very peaceful.

"I'm happy that he appeared to have slept through the whole ordeal," she commented.

"It seems he did so."

Although Guy has attended The Little Paradise Child Care for only six months, he has certainly felt at home with them. He doesn't cry whenever he's dropped off by his parents. He sleeps very well and doesn't seem to pick up any illness from them. His language power has rather developed very fast. He has also made several friends and their staff seemed to have accepted him as their own.

As their car was a few metres from the main entrance gate of the Child Care Centre, they spotted Mrs Christy Botsile, the owner and Matron in charge who appeared to be stepping out of her office door and subsequently appeared to be heading to the gate.

Abigail peered ahead, "Is Mrs Botsile coming to open the gate for us?"

"It seems so," Sammy responded. "Is it because Bandile the gate man isn't on duty to open the gate today?"

"Or could she just be excited because of Guy's birthday ceremony?" Abigail questioned.

Sammy observed, "It could be all of the above."

They both chuckled.

By the time their car got to the gate Mrs Botsile had already come outside the gate to welcome them.

"How did you escape the rioters?" she asked.

Sammy wound down his window, "We were just lucky."

Mrs Botsile is a tall, very attractive black woman from Soweto. She is the quintessence of beauty. She could still make the front page of a play-boy magazine if she chooses to. She was said to have been a model in her hay days. Her face has eyes well seated in their sockets like a perfect sculpture. Her voice has a soothing effect to it which usually acts as a lullaby not only to men around her but also to the kids in her care. Her dark unwrinkled olive skin hides her true 45 years of existence. Under the breeze her brown curly hair fluffs around like kids dancing in the moonlight. She has no children of her own, having suffered several miscarriages, most of which occurred due to the domestic violence she suffered at the hands of her previous husband. She was attracted and trapped in the marriage for economic reasons having come from a very poor background. Her husband who was some 15 years older than her was very unpredictable. He accused her of infidelity and was very physical with her.

In South Africa women are killed every day by their partners or lovers. She ran away from him and began divorce proceedings while being in hiding. She did so before he was able to send her to the great beyond. Her new husband is 10 years younger than her and happy to be with her even though she has no children. It is her love for children that compelled her to create the Child Care Centre.

She approached the passenger's car door and opened it, "Birthday boy, come to me," Mrs Botsile announced and helped Guy to climb down from the car.

She pressed the remote key and the gate opened. "You can drive through," she encouraged Sammy and Abigail. She too walked back in with Guy by her side.

Sammy and Abigail drove their car into the compound and then stepped out. "Are we alone?" Sammy asked.

"Other kids and parents are already around. A few more are yet to arrive, and we fear they may not get through because of the riots," Mrs Botsile concluded.

Walking behind Mrs Botsile and Guy, Abigail asked, "How many are here?"

Mrs Botsile halted briefly to allow Abigail and Sammy to catch up with them. "15 kids and their parents have arrived."

They walked into the large room, which is Mrs Botsile's office. Adjacent to Mrs Botsile's rooms, one gets into the first room designated for 0 – 2 years, then into the rooms for older kids.

Sammy had been here a number of times but still finds himself trapped in the exquisite beauty that the rooms exude. He can't help himself as he glances from one room to the other with keen interest and admiration, pacing around them speechlessly.

The Child Care Centre is intended for children from an upper echelon of society. Its buildings are next to none in beauty and decorations. They were designed with a climate friendly touch. There are three separate rooms although adjoined. Each room is specially designed to cater for a specific age ranges from 0 -2 years, 2 – 4 years, and 4 – 6 years. There are five small beds aligned close to each room, and at another end of the room a playground with assorted toys. There is a toilet and change room attached to each room. The walls of each room are brightly coloured and are dominated by a design or some other form of artistry work from ancient to modern. There are sculptures in the older kids' rooms, paintings of Nelson Mandela and Winnie Mandela in others, freelance drawings and plain visual arts in others. Suddenly he felt a hand on his shoulder as he was engrossed with the painting of Mona Lisa. "Darling the ceremony is about to start," Abigail whispers into his ears.

"Oh, okay." He was brought back to reality by his wife. "Let's get going."

Hand in hand, they both walked into Mrs Botsile's office and took Guy from the sofa where he was sleeping and through the foyer to the outside where people sat under the canopies.

There were three canopies. Two had a well decorated table with 10 chairs and 10 high chairs. Drums and other music instruments were located in the third canopy. Each of the tables had a vase of flowers in the middle. The second canopy had a neon party light decoration in it. There was a microphone standing in front of the middle canopy.

The choice of the spot couldn't have been better. The colour of canopy was bluish with yellowish strips in the middle. The grass had been mowed so low that the ground showed its beauty through it. It could pass for artificial carpet grass. Gentle breezes were blowing and well-cut hedges and grasses around the Childcare Centre were moving in steady synchronised waves as though dancing to some well-orchestrated music being sung by the birds that perched in the surrounding trees.

"Hello Aby." Abigail and Sammy look in the direction of the voice. "Your seat is here," Merci advised. "I'll be with you shortly." She informed them and went to attend to others.

Merci Mang is Abigail's neighbour and the Second in command in this Child Care Centre. She and her partner recommended the Centre to Abigail and Sammy. They make their way to the middle canopy and sit down.

Abigail's eyes strayed to the roof of the canopies and through their crevices she gazed into the blue sky and lapsed into memory lane...

∞ ∞

She imagined the Creator as a great artist who designed the ever-changing colours of the sky with the clouds which were transformed into infinite images of beauty. The clouds were on great display; most were thin and velvety. The thicker ones were a whitish colour which were convoluted and drifted into some serene views on one side thus forming the beautiful images of horse's heads at one end and in their middle they formed ships filled with white sails and far away they merged into the forget-me-not blueness of the sky. It's the Universe's great display at its very best.

Serenity appeared to descend from the sky into Abigail's mind. She felt a sense of contentment and fulfilment and a feeling of deep gratitude knowing that she now had a baby who had undergone gene manipulation, thanks to the IVF program that was organised by Drs OsGood and DoLittle. The calmness of the sky was reflected in the calmness of her mind, knowing that her child would never suffer from epilepsy and wouldn't' go through what Mighty M (her late father-in-law) went through. And at worst wouldn't die in a bathtub!

"Were you caught up in the riots this morning?" Merci asked and that brought Abigail back to reality.

"Yeah, we were," she affirmed.

Abigail straightened Guy's neck which was dangling out of her shoulder like a fruit out of a tree branch.

"Did you suffer any injury or damage to any of your belongings?" Merci asked.

"Not really. We were extricated from the middle of it all by a Police escort."

"I was also lucky but my niece wasn't that lucky."

Upon hearing that somebody had suffered some harm, Sammy became interested in the ladies' discussion. "So, what happened to her?" he asked.

"Well, it was largely her own problem; she was one of the rioters and suffered some eye damage when she was hit with the Police tear gas."

"Oh, that's not too good," exclaimed Abigail. "Was she taken to the hospital?"

"Yeah, she was. She has actually been moved from one hospital to another?"

"Why, what was the problem?" Sammy enquired.

"They state that she reacted to the tear gas in an abnormal way. The doctors have advised that she has an immune deficiency which makes it difficult for her system to dissolve the chemicals in the tear gas."

Abigail's eyes became dilated. "Does it mean that she'll go blind?"

"It's possible."

As they were conversing, the Master of Ceremony tapped the microphone in a bid to get everyone's attention, and then began, "Hello ladies, gentlemen and kids, welcome to today's birthday ceremony." He paused as people were still conversing. He tapped the microphone again. "I'm DJ Andy. Today's event is all about our little Guy Petters. We're here to celebrate his first birthday."

As Andy was talking, Guy woke up and stepped out of his mother's arms. He ran out into the foyer and through Mrs Botsile's room.

Abigail ran after him and grabbed him. "Come and stay with mummy," she pleaded with him and Guy rushed into her arms and they both went back to the table.

On their arrival, DJ Andy asked, "Do you mind if the neon party light is switched on?"

Abigail consented. "Sure, you can do so."

The middle canopy light displayed Guy's name as it flickered from one colour to another. It was very close to where Guy sat with his parents.

DJ Andy continued, "We shall sing a happy birthday song for the celebrant; get him to cut the cake, take pictures ..." He paused as he noticed that Guy was not looking so good.

Guy's eyes rolled then he vomited and his arms and legs began to jerk.

Sammy leapt from his chair and grabbed Guy from Abigail and laid him on the floor until the seizure subsided.

Abigail began to cry and scream.

Mrs Botsile immediately ran into her office and returned in a few minutes. A short while later, a middle-aged man rushed into the building with a stethoscope around his neck.

"Where's the child?" he asked.

Mrs Botsile pointed to Guy who was now on his father's lap still appearing very weak and sleepy.

Mrs Botsile approached Sammy, "This is Doctor Joshua. His clinic is in the next building. We use him if we need urgent medical attention." She paused briefly. "Hope you people don't mind. I called him."

Dr Joshua reached for Guy while he was still in Sammy's arms. "What's your name Sir?"

"I'm Sammy." He pointed to his left, "She's Abigail and is my wife. My son's name is Guy."

Dr Joshua began to examine Guy while Mrs Botsile and Merci dismissed every other guest including DJ Andy.

After the general examination, Dr Joshua checked Guy's temperature and reported, "It's 37.8 degrees Celsius."

Abigail had calmed down now. "It means he has slight temperature?" She asked.

"You're correct."

"Could the rise in temperature cause him to have a convulsion?" Abigail asked. She favoured convulsion rather than seizure. Mighty M had seizures. Guy will not.

"It's a possibility. Other things are also possible," replied Dr Joshua. "We need an ambulance and get him to the hospital right now."

Abigail clinched her fists. "We would prefer to be transferred to Pretoria Hospital where we have family members."

"Okay, we shall do that right away." Dr Joshua replied and stepped aside to make some phone calls.

While he was doing that, Sammy rang Uncle Goddy. "We're coming to Pretoria in the next few hours."

"Why, what's the matter?" Uncle Goddy asked.

In between sobbing, "Guy has had a seizure," he replied.

"Oh, what a mess?" Uncle Goddy exclaimed. "Okay, I'll make the necessary contacts and arrangements with Life Matters Best Hospital."

"Thanks Uncle. You're the best!" Sammy praised him.

As Sammy was concluding his discussion with Uncle Goddy, the ambulance vehicle drove in through the gate.

Two men who were wearing the *Paramedics On Call Ambulance* Service uniform stepped out.

Dr Joshua described the situation to them and they then approached Sammy and Abigail and introduced themselves as Nick and Edwards.

"How's Guy doing now?" Nick asked.

"He's weak but can be aroused."

Nick quickly checked Guy and put him on the stretcher, then into the ambulance.

Sammy and Abigail turned around to Mrs Botsile, Dr Joshua and Merci and thanked them. They then climbed into the ambulance with their son and the vehicle left the Little Paradise Child Care for Life Matters Best Hospital in Pretoria.

Chapter 13

Room 5
Paediatric Ward
Life Matters Best Hospital
No 40 Georgina Avenue
Groenkloof 0281, Pretoria
South Africa
September 22, 1990, Saturday Evening

"How's Guy doing now?" Uncle Goddy asked as he hobbled as fast as his weak limp would carry him, into Guy's Paediatric room.

Looking distraught and disheartened Abigail replied, "He had two convulsions while we were in the ambulance."

"One was full, and the other was mini ..." her husband corrected her.

"We contacted you because we wanted to come back as we believe this is where the children specialists are. We need answers as to what is happening to him." Abigail sounded frustrated.

"I made all the phone calls after I had the discussion with Sammy," Uncle Goddy replied. He then began to hobble from one end of the room to the other. "Has he been reviewe?"

"No, he hasn't been seen by a doctor yet,"she held her breath then continued. "Several nurses have been in and out of here like bees visiting the honey site."

Sammy chipped in to correct Abigail, "An intern, I think that's what they're called, breezed in and announced that she was going to bring the specialist in, then left. She has not come back since then."

Uncle Goddy was irked, "This is a sick child and should take pre-eminence. More so, we're private paying patients and should be reviewed quickly."

He doesn't know why a doctor hasn't come around to see him yet.

Sammy sat in a coiled position with his face on his knees. "They say he's stable," he mumbled.

"I'll go and fetch a goddamn doctor now," Uncle Goddy vouched and stormed out.

Sammy's muscles began to tighten in spasms of fear. He's not known to give in to such emotions. He believes he's stoic. But his nerves are failing him now. His own child, his flesh and blood, is lying helpless on the bed. Is this epilepsy or a convulsion as the doctor that they saw in the Child Care Centre had suggested? Only the doctors here, specialists they are called, will know. They'll do tests and they will confirm.

Fear began to crawl through Sammy's muscles to his heart, and to his head. Fear of the unknown, fear of the worst scenario eventuating and most probably nameless fear. It travelled through Sammy's veins and made its way into his brain. His brain ceased to function. As his eyes darted from Guy's head to his toes he couldn't make out if he was breathing normally or about to begin to have another attack. The more he tried to register what his eyes were seeing, the more he failed. His brain was functioning like a mobile phone that was within a mountain range – out of range or at best having poor reception. But he remained calm or at least believed he was so. He used his cupped hand to cover his mouth and nostril to disguise his rapid and shallow breathing. His shoes kept his toenails from creating holes in the floor. His stomach felt knotted up and his pulse pounded away.

Silence and fear gripped him and lingered in his head creating an eerie atmosphere.

At that time he noticed Uncle Goddy walked back in with a slim tall young man who had a stethoscope round his neck.

The doctor was talking to Uncle Goddy and Abigail. Sammy was in trance and largely uninterested. He was in a world of his own.

In a split second his eyes darted from Guy to his Abigail who was tilting out of her chair and heading to the ground.

"Gee, she is falling," he screamed and rushed to her side.

Abigail had been listening to the doctor but registering nothing. Her eyes couldn't be shifted away from the tiny body of Guy. She now had more wrinkles than her mother. She wore a worried look and couldn't fathom out what the hell was going on in their life.

She couldn't even register the doctor's name. The more the doctor spoke, the more distanced she became. She'd had gene manipulation and IVF through the best hospital and couldn't fault the procedure from start to finish. They gave her 99% assurance that all went well. But here she was with Guy being very ill.

She looked up again and tried to focus on the doctor. Abigail didn't like the doctor. He spoke too fast and too confidently. He was slim and tall and had long blond hair. He looked too handsome. The more she watched him, the more he reminded her of Henry, her first love. She met Henry when she was barely 16. She was in a blissful relationship. Two years into the relationship, Henry had a motor cycle accident and died. She couldn't forgive him to this day because he defied her advice not to go on the so-call dirt-ride competition.

"Snap out of this," Abigail told herself. But the more she tried, the more she saw Henry in front of her. 'It seems I'm having a dream,' she told herself and vigorously shook her head to wake up.

"Hello Henry, how are you?" she heard herself mutter.

Geraldine, Sammy's mum rushed to Abigail's side and wedged herself between her and the ground.

"Lower her to the ground," the doctor commanded. "And then position her on her left side."

Geraldine did as she was told. By the time Abigail was on the ground three nurses clenching different types of apparatus came flying in.

The doctor knelt down beside Abigail and tapped her on the shoulder. "Hello, Mrs Petters, how're you? Open your eyes."

As the doctor was examining her, Abigail slowly opened her eyes.

The face of Sammy, his mother, Uncle Goddy and every other person in the room lit up immediately she opened her eyes.

The doctor looked up at his nurses. "Emma, please can you check her BP and heart rate."

"Yes, Dr Lucas," Nurse Emma replied and began to apply the BP cuff on her arm.

"Eva, please set up face mask and let 12 litres of oxygen run in."

"Will do," Nurse Eva replied and began to connect the oxygen cylinder and the face mask.

Dr Lucas then turned to the last nurse who was waiting for her own instructions. "Isabella, please grab a bag of saline and advise the porter to bring another bed for her." He took a deep breath and quickly scanned Abigail. "She may need it."

Dr Lucas returned his attention to the sick lady on the ground. "Mrs Petters, do you want to get up to the bed?" he asked.

Abigail nodded.

Dr Lucas looked at Nurse Eva, "Remove the mask from her face."

Abigail then began to wipe away the tears that were streaming down her cheeks. As she cleared the tears away, she blinked several times, glancing at everyone in the room with some level of concentration. As she glanced around, she moved her eyebrows down and closer together and clinched her teeth in a way to reassure herself that she was back to land of the living.

She gradually reached out to Sammy's hand that then helped her to rise. Immediately she was upright she shut her eyes momentarily like she was trying to erase the image of herself on the ground. Her hand reached into her handbag which was lying nearby, and she grabbed her handkerchief and dabbed her eyes several times.

"Are you okay?" Uncle Goddy asked.

"Yeah, I am." Abigail replied.

"She's okay," Dr Lucas confirmed.

Abigail looked askance at Sammy, "What happened to me?"

Sammy looked at Dr Lucas as if he was seeking the doctor to bail him out.

The doctor got the gist. "You faintly briefly—in medicine we call it vaso-vagal syncope," he advised her.

With her legs still quivering, Abigail slowly lowered herself onto the edge of the bed where Guy lay. She took a deep breath. "So, I lost consciousness."

"Yes, you did but it was only momentarily." Dr Lucas reassured her. "It tends to happen to some people when they're exposed to an overwhelming event."

Sammy looked concerned. "Do you mean that our son's condition could've triggered her collapse?"

"Exactly so," Dr Lucas affirmed.

Sammy grinned and shook his head. He focussed squarely on Dr Lucas, "She mentioned Henry—an old boyfriend—before she collapsed, how do we relate that to the child's convulsions?"

The doctor hesitated briefly before speaking. "It would have been like an apparition. She would've seen a figure that was not there."

Neither Sammy nor Abigail pursued the discussion any further.

Dr Lucas was concerned that Abigail might lapse into a coma, and pointing to the bed that was just rolled into the room, "Why don't you make yourself comfortable on the other bed?"

Abigail, with slight staggering steps and with Sammy's support, moved over to the new bed. She lay on her back, stared briefly at the ceiling before shutting her eyes.

Sammy stared at limp body of Guy on the bed and noticing some slight limb movements. "It seems that he's beginning to twitch." He turned to Dr Lucas for reassurance.

Dr Lucas quickly drew closer to the bed, placed his stethoscope on Guy's chest. As he was doing that Guy's right arm began to swing forward and backward.

"Get me Midazolam," Dr Lucas quietly instructed Nurse Eva.

Nurse Eva walked over to the other side of the room, pulled out a drawer in the trolley and dipped her hand into the drug box, grabbing an ampoule of Midazolam. She then brought out a syringe and aspirated the content of the ampoule into it. "Here it is," she announced to the doctor.

Doctor Lucas spread out his hand, collected it and looked at the ampoule. "Hope you've checked its expiry date?"

"It's in date." Nurse Eva confirmed.

At this time, both Guy's limbs had begun to do the rhythmic jerking motions, his eyes had also begun to roll upwards and he was producing foams.

Noticing what is happening; everyone rose to their feet, Abigail leaped out of her bed and ran to Guy. Sammy stopped her before she was able to reach him.

Doctor Lucas was attending to Guy. He calmly rolled Guy onto his side. "Put oxygen on him. Set it up at 8 litres please," he ordered.

Nurse Eva nodded and began to couple the oxygen onto the mask.

As Nurse Eva was fixing the oxygen mask to Guy's face, Dr Lucas began to inject the Midazolam into his right thigh. Then he inserted a cannula and collected blood. "Emma, can we grab this boy's vital signs please?"

"Temperature is 37.8 degrees, respiratory rate is 25, and heart rate 110 and his saturation is 99 percent," Nurse Emma announced.

Dr Lucas completed a laboratory form for some bloods to be done. "Nurse Eva, please take these to the lab." He then handed both the blood he collected and the lab form to her. She left the room quickly.

Some minutes later, Guy calmed down and went into a deep sleep.

The remaining two nurses then requested to be allowed to go back to their duty posts and to attend to other patients.

"Sure, you can go. I'll let you know if I need you people again," Dr Lucas told them.

They began to march out of the room one by one, as they came. Nurse Emma was the last to leave. As she was on the door, Dr Lucas watched her for some moments then suddenly bellowed out, "Please

Nurse Emma, will you remember to come back and check Guy's temperature in an hour's time to ensure that it hasn't skyrocketed."

Nurse Emma turned around, gave him a smile and nodded in acquiescence.

Abigail wished to bring Dr Lucas' attention back to Guy, "Dr Lucas, he urinated himself while he was fitting." Abigail reported and raised Guy's nappies which she has just taken out for him to see.

Dr Lucas edged slightly forward from where he was and looked at Guy's nappies on Abigail's hand. "It's common for that to happen in both febrile seizures and in epilepsy."

"Are these fits or seizures, and are they due to febrile illness as you pointed out?" Abigail paused. "Or are they due to epilepsy?"

"Actually, fits and seizures mean the same thing and can be used inter-changeably."

Sammy decided to step in. "We want to confirm if it's likely that he's having epileptic fits."

Dr Lucas felt like a thunderbolt had hit him. He was taken unaware by the question. He took a breath and slowly lowered his huge frame onto a chair. He appeared flabbergasted by Sammy's question or at least thrown off balance by it.

He looked squarely at Sammy, "My response will be two-fold – first I'll make an effort to explain febrile convulsion and epilepsy to you people and secondly, I'll ask you to tell me why you want to know." He stopped and threw a glance across the room from Sammy, through Abigail to other people in the room including Uncle Goddy and Geraldine.

"Fits in children…," he cleared his throat, "are usually due to febrile convulsion except if they're persisting or there are reasons to assume otherwise."

"Our son's seizures have become recurrent, haven't they?" asked Sammy.

"It seems so. He had two while in the ambulance and one here."

Abigail's eyes squinted, "So, does it mean that his are no longer febrile seizures?"

"No, I've not said so. He has had a raised temperature which will still compel us to consider febrile convulsion in this instance, except ..."

Abigail barged in, not allowing him to complete his sentence, "For the fact that we've significant family history of epilepsy."

Dr Lucas' eyes lit up immediately. "What exactly do you mean by significant family history?"

"My father-in-law died from it."

"Okay, I get it."

Sammy had gone to ease himself. He came back into the room and had overheard the discussion. "Doctor, will you be confident to tell us that Guy has epilepsy now?"

"No, I won't be, because febrile convulsion is rife in children between the ages of six months and five years. Your son is only 12 months old."

"Could he also have epilepsy?" asked Abigail.

"Yes, it's possible if there's any other serious underlying health issue..."

"Underlying health issue like what?" Abigail asked.

"Epilepsy is a possibility because of your family history but that will become relevant when he is older than five years."

Abigail immediately sat up and looked at Dr Lucas. "We manipulated his gene in order to get rid of the epilepsy."

"Who did that for you, and in which hospital?"

"It was organised by Drs OsGood and DoLittle and in your hospital, the Out Reach Clinic in Bloemfontein," Abigail responded.

Dr Lucas immediately grabbed his phone from his pocket, "It means that we could get your file if I search our system here."

"Yes, you should."

Dr Lucas dialled their Medical Records, and they heard him say, "Hello Henrietta, please print out copies of the electronic file of Mr Sammy Petters DOB: 02/02/1960 and Mrs Abigail Petters DOB: 05/06/1960 and send them to me in Paediatric Room 5 as soon as possible."

"Consider it done," they heard Henrietta respond.

"Please search their files in the Out Reach section," he concluded.

Within five minutes of making the call they heard a knock on the door.

A young lady in her early 20s walked in, "Here's the file, Sir." She then handed two files to him.

Dr Lucas took the files from her, "Thanks Henrietta," he muttered as he began to flip through them. Henrietta left the room.

Dr Lucas continued to go through the files and appeared deeply absorbed in the contents. Abigail's question forced him to look up. "We're worried and concerned that the gene manipulation might have failed given the seizures that Guy is having."

"I won't draw such conclusions yet." Dr Lucas said trying to reassure them.

Uncle Goddy tapped Sammy on the shoulder, "Do you mind if I ask him to read what Dr OsGood and his team did?"

"Not at all. Go ahead."

"Hello Dr Lucas, can you please read out or give us a summary of what the gene manipulation involved."

Dr Lucas began, "From the content of the file, Dr OsGood was assisted by Dr DoLittle. They took your sperm Mr Petters, and eggs from you Mrs Petters, and then proceeded to perform an in vitro fertilisation with the eggs and sperm they collected." He looked at Sammy. "Is that correct?"

"Absolutely so."

Abigail also nodded in acceptance.

Dr Lucas then continued, "Then they used CRISPR/Cas7 to edit the genomes of the embryos. The editing targeted a GABRA1 gene which specifically involves ion-channel." He glanced at Uncle Goddy and the others seeking to confirm that they were following him.

Uncle Goddy gave him thumbs up.

"They then inserted the embryo after the gene manipulation into you, Mrs Petters, and you went on to deliver Guy. Is that right?"

Abigail agreed. "What's the relevance of GABRA1 gene?"

"It's inherited in an autosomal dominant pattern, which means one copy of the altered gene in each cell is sufficient to cause the disorder. Another important gene which they didn't mention if they isolated and treated was EFHCI gene which is involved in juvenile myoclonic epilepsy or other forms of epilepsy in a way that is not clearly known to us."

By this time Abigail was raging with anger. She was not sure if her anger would be directed to Dr OsGood or to Dr Lucas who was now casting doubts on the gene manipulation which they'd believed was very successful. She now knew why she hated Dr Lucas from the onset. He is just like Henry; that guy she'd dated back in Teacher's training school who was sleek and untrustworthy filthy liar. She couldn't help but to blurt out, "Do you mean that the gene manipulation was not successful because of the lack of treatment of the EFHCI gene?"

"You'll know in a few years to come," was Dr Lucas reply.

At that instance, Guy began to fit again, and Dr Lucas pressed the red button and the nurses rushed in. He advised them to give him Midazolam and to organise an EEG, and MRI.

Epilogue

With deep concern and desire to get rid of epilepsy which killed his father, Sammy and his wife, Abigail set out to arrange for gene manipulation so that their unborn child will not have any trace of epilepsy in his system.

Guy was the product of the gene manipulation. He showed no signs of seizure from birth until he was 12 months old when he had a massive seizure.

Was the gene manipulation successful?

Follow us in Part Two for answers…

Made in United States
Orlando, FL
05 November 2026

90275227R00083